Mental Health Interventions for the Aging

Mental Health Interventions for the Aging

Arthur MacNeill Horton, Jr.
and Contributors

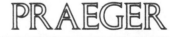

PRAEGER SPECIAL STUDIES • PRAEGER SCIENTIFIC
A J.F. BERGIN PUBLISHERS BOOK

Library of Congress Cataloging in Publication Data
Main entry under title:

Mental health interventions for the aging.

Includes bibliographies and index.
1. Geriatric psychiatry.   2. Psychotherapy—In old age.
I. Horton, Arthur MacNeill, 1947-   [DNLM: WT 150 M5494]IS
RC451.4.A5M455   618.97'689   81-10176
ISBN 0-03—061607-7   AACR2

All rights reserved by J.F. Bergin Publishers, Inc.
670 Amherst Road
South Hadley, Massachusetts 01075

Published in 1982 by Praeger Publishers
CBS Educational and Professional Publishing
A Division of CBS, Inc.
521 Fifth Avenue, New York, New York 10175

0 056 987654321

Printed in the United States of America

Contents

v

Preface

Perhaps one of the most salient concerns of contemporary health care is the eminent explosive growth of the elderly population in America. Demographic and epidemiological data are non-controversial on this point. Factors such as an extended life expectancy and the post-World War II baby boom clearly imply the need for increased attention to the problems of the aged. Current census data suggests that the proportion of the population over sixty-five—twenty-two to twenty-three million or 19%, at present—will double by the year 2030. In the United States today there are more nursing home beds than acute care hospital beds. While up to one half of all nursing home residents may have personal and emotional adjustment problems, psychotherapeutic treatment is more often unavailable or nonexistant for this population. As mental health emerges as a full participant in the health care delivery system, a greater focus upon treatment approaches to the elderly would appear inevitable.

This book was organized in order to highlight this developing area of clinical and research interest. The chapters were solicited to provide contrasting viewpoints on the multifaceted interaction of the geriatric individual, his/her environment, and his/her behavior. Contributions include discussions of both time-honored methods of psychotherapeutic intervention and a number of rather innovative approaches to positive behavior change.

The introductory chapter places the psychotherapy of the aged within the context of human behavior changes and briefly discusses clinical neuropsychological assessment of elderly individuals. Traditional approaches are usually classified as individual psychotherapy and group psychotherapy with geriatric individuals. Separate chapters on each of these psychotherapeutic modalities have been included, in addition to chapters on approaches which have evolved more recently. Generally speaking, these approaches have a more specialized focus. Separate chapters on habitability (the design of special environments for the elderly), rehabilitation of the neurologically impaired aged, reality orientation, geriatric bibliotherapy, and behavior therapy with the elderly have been included to introduce the readers to new methods which will have a predictable,enduring influence upon the psychotherapeutic treatment of the aging. In order to provide some conceptual integration of the contrasting viewpoints on interactions of the geriatric individual, a commentary chapter has been contributed. The primary focus of the discussion is the ability of mental health professionals to contribute adequate, innovative solutions to the human welfare problems of the aged. Also, a critical evaluation of the contemporary knowledge base necessary for attempting meaningful geriatric mental health interventions is undertaken and the issue of appropriate interface with society's traditional systems of socialization and support with this age group is addressed.

This book has been designed for a broad interdisciplinary audience. Given the real need for a single reference which will provide a basic overview of psychotherapeutic treatment strategies with the aged, it is expected that individuals from a wide variety of backgrounds will find it helpful. The readership may range from social work trainees to psychiatric residents. This is well, and as it should be, for individuals from many different professional orientations will need to contribute their enthusiasm, encouragement, and expertise in order for all of us to even begin to cope with the mental health problems of the aged. The expectation and hope is that delineation of these concerns will be of some value in meeting the challenge of alleviating human distress and promoting social well-being for the elderly population.

Arthur MacNeill Horton, Jr.

Mental Health
Interventions
for the Aging

1

Introduction to the Psychotherapy of the Aging

Arthur MacNeill Horton, Jr.

Any discussion of psychotherapy for older individuals must first deal with the well-publicized views of Freud (1950). During a lecture, in 1904, Freud stated that:

> The age of patients has this importance in determining their fitness for psycho-analytic treatment; that, on the one hand, near or above the fifties, the elasticity of mental processes, on which the treatment depends, is as a rule lacking—older people are no longer educable—and, on the other hand, the mass of material to be dealt with would prolong the duration of treatment indefinitely. (Freud 1950 pp. 258-259)

It might be observed that this rather pessimistic perspective has been quite influential with mental health workers. As summarized by Garfield, the popular view of the elderly as candidates for psychotherapy is relatively unchanged:

> It has generally been assumed that older people tend to be more rigid and fixed in their ways. Their patterns of behavior have a longer reinforcement history and supposedly their defences and character structure are more resistant to decline in mental functioning (Wechsler 1958), and that they may not learn new skills as readily as younger in-

This chapter was written by Arthur MacNeill Horton, Jr. in his private capacity. No official support or endorsement by the Veterans Administration is intended or should be inferred.

dividuals. Consequently, it could be presumed that they would be less favorable candidates for psychotherapy in terms of their potential for change. (Garfield 1978, p. 212)

While the acceptance of the opinion of an authority is both a traditional and a popular approach to knowledge, it should be noted that tradition and popularity are flawed approaches to truth. With regard to the unsuitability of the elderly as candidates for psychotherapy, for example, there is a dearth of solid research evidence (Garfield 1978). While some would contend that classical psychoanalysis of an older adult may require too many years to be practically contemplated, the research data do not support the view that older clients are less desirable in terms of other psychotherapeutic approaches (Garfield 1978). Indeed, a review of the scientific literature on age and psychotherapeutic outcome by Luborsky, Chandler, Auerbach, Cohen, and Bachrach (1971) appeared to find no clear-cut relationships. Thus, it would be inappropriate to form negative conclusions. Perhaps the most sound advice is the following suggestion by Garfield:

One should not discuss age in relation to outcome in the abstract, but instead should specify a particular age in relation to a particular therapy and with full awareness of the other possible factors that may play a role in outcome. (Garfield 1978, p. 213)

The present chapter, therefore, will present an introduction to the psychotherapy of the elderly that focuses upon the interactive nature of age and therapy. First, an examination of the special characteristics, life change and mental health needs of the elderly will be discussed. Second, an admittedly superficial over-view of the psychotherapeutic process will be presented. Third, possible future directions in psychotherapy with particular relevance to the elderly will be outlined. While the limitations of space require relatively cursory treatment of these important topics, still these introductory remarks may serve to provide a framework for better appreciation of the other more specialized chapters in this volume.

CHARACTERISTICS OF THE AGED

There is rather strong evidence that the number of older adults in the United States is increasing. Current census data suggests that the proportion of the population over the age sixty-five (twenty-two to twenty-three million or 19% at present) will double by the year 2030 (U.S. Department of Commerce 1977). Given that the numbers of the aged are increasing dramatically, the question arises: How are they different as a group from younger individuals?

Developmental Changes

Physical. One gerontologist, in a semi-serious mood, suggested that there are a number of simple ways for younger people to experience the physical changes that the aged undergo. Quite simply, one needs to smear vasoline over one's glasses, put rocks in one's shoes and cotton in one's ears, then put on rubber gloves. This sounds fairly goulish but is probably somewhat accurate.

There are definite physical changes which occur with aging. A good many of these are obvious from simple observation of one's self or one's relatives. For example, baldness, graying of the hair, a decline in physical stature, wrinkling, dryness, and sagging of the skin, diminution of secondary sexual characteristics and muscular tone as well as muscular bulk are all so much a part of every day life, that one almost forgets to think of them.

Other changes are less amenable to visual observation. For example, visceral changes such as atrophy of the testes, liver, lungs, and kidneys, are attributable to aging. In addition, there are central nervous system changes; i.e., loss of cells in the nervous system occurs in the human neocortex with aging (Brody 1955). All in all, physical strength and the ability to do manual labor declines among those of advanced age (Hurlock 1968).

Sensory. Similar to changes in physical abilities sensory abilities also decline with increasing age. Vision is less efficient as the pupil size of the eye diminishes with age. Both the abilities to discern small details and to perceive color decrease with advancing age. Because of this, older individuals require increased illumination. Hearing, also, decreases with age. The major losses, however, are for the higher frequencies (Telford and Sawrey 1977). Thus, general conversational speech can still be understood. In addition, sensitivity to pain decreases with age. The loss of pain sensitivity becomes most sailent after age sixty (Schulderman and Zubek 1962).

Mental. As a general rule, the performance of individuals on standard intelligence tests decreases as they age (Telford and Sawrey 1977). At the same time, these changes may not be as serious as has been popularly assumed (Baltes and Labourie 1973). Indeed, some would assert that the intellectual aging in current cohorts is much more plastic and heterogeneous than previously thought (Willis and Baltes 1980). One of many issues involved in this discussion is, of course, the relevance of intelligence tests developed to assess academic potential of school children for predicting the day to day functioning of their grandparents.

Interestingly, a recent review of neuropsychological test results for aging individuals (Horton 1980) supports the view that abilities which involve immediate novel problem solving and particularly preceptual-motor or psychomotor responding are most effected while those abilities which are dependent upon relatively automatic and overlearned abilities, such as vocabulary or the recall of general information are less effected.

Life Changes

Quite clearly, the advancing years produce many rather profound life changes for the elderly. Among others, retirement, sexual role, and social status all undergo modification. Retirement brings the loss of a familiar working environment and the problem of filling many empty hours. Compounding these difficulties is the loss of income.

Sexual activity among the aged is an area rife with myth. Research results have documented that the aged may be sexually active until their seventies despite popular attitudes to the contrary (Telford and Sawrey 1977). Indeed, there are those who would suggest that intercourse has a therapeutic value with the aged (Horn 1974). The problem, however, is dealing with a lack of sex partners, in the event of a death of a spouse, and the attitudes of others.

Social status changes are also sources of stress for the elderly. For example, the losses of social interaction with children and the parent role, the possible death of a spouse and the absence of a defined occupational position all may contribute to emotional dissatisfaction. The previously discussed developmental changes in physical, sensory, and mental abilities can only be seen as augmenting social status changes.

Mental Health Needs

As one would expect from the above paragraphs, elderly individuals are a population in need of mental health services. Various review articles have reported estimates of the need for services. Kramer, Tauke, and Redick (1973) suggested that 10% to 20% of persons age sixty-five or older were in need of mental health services. Among a number of serious problems, two which might be mentioned specifically are depression and senile dementia (or organic brain syndrome). Butler and Lewis (1977) found that depression is the most common psychiatric complaint among older adults. As is well known, there is a high rate of suicide among older adults.

Similarly, senile dementia is a serious mental health hazard for the elderly. Interestingly, organic brain disorders account for 38.12% of all patient care episodes for patients over the age of sixty-five (Horton 1980). Rather startling is the fact that the current mental health system is bereft of adequate programs to identify and serve older adults with organic brain syndrome (Gatz, Smyer, and Lawton 1980).

In the next section of this chapter, an introduction to psychotherapy will be provided. As following chapters will discuss a number of different psychotherapeutic approaches with the aging in some detail, this overview of psychotherapeutic process will be somewhat rudimentary and will concentrate upon constituted elements of psychotherapy. Specific applications to the aging will come in the later chapters in this volume.

AN OVERVIEW OF PSYCHOTHERAPY

An old hospital saying defines psychotherapy as "a blanket that covers many sins." and there appears to be a certain amount of truth in this definition. Psychotherapy, as it is currently practiced, is a remarkably heterogeneous process. Included under its aegis are psychoanalytic sessions which last for years, biofeedback sessions that last for minutes, progressive relaxation training, primal scream therapy, psychodrama, and marathon encounter groups. Perhaps one usable definition would be:

> Psychotherapy is an interpersonal process designed to bring about modification of feelings, cognitions, attitudes, and behavior which have proven troublesome to the person seeking help from a trained professional (Strupp 1978, p. 3).

While admittedly leaving many gaps, this definition at least provides some sort of direction as to the purpose of psychotherapeutic endeavor. In order to provide a better understanding of the essential elements of psychotherapy, Kiesler (1971) proposed a grid model to delineate the crucial variables (that is, the major constructs components of the psychotherapeutic endeavor can be delineated as relatively few constructs). These are patient, treatment, and therapist variables. Each will be discussed in turn.

Patients

Perhaps the most obvious fact is that different patients will have different effects on which method of psychotherapy is used and how it is carried out. It must again be stressed, however, that age is not a determinant. The classic division of patients on a continuum was proposed by Schofield (1964). He proposed that therapists preferred to work with the "YAVIS" patient: patients who are young, attractive, verbal, intelligent, and successful. An example of this sort of patient would be a blond college cheerleader, of the opposite sex, and a 3.8 average, majoring in speech and drama, coming to a university counseling center to discuss a complaint of pervasive anxiety. The other end of the spectrum is the "HOUND" patient, homely, old, unattractive, nonverbal and dumb. An example of this sort of patient is the elderly schizophrenic who had difficulty in the third grade, is functionally illiterate, speaks in monosyllables and bears a striking resemblance to Quasimodo. Given the two possible extremes and the human nature of therapists, it is fairly straightforward as to who is more likely to be seen for extended sessions.

While the "YAVIS-HOUND" continuum is helpful in giving an overview and appears in line with research on patient improvement (Garfield 1978), a more heuristic structure would be to consider a simplified model of psychopathology. The number of disorders and conditions a comprehensive discussion of psychopathology would require is beyond the scope of this book. Kroger and Folger (1976) discuss twenty-five different categories of complaints to be treated by psychotherapy.

So in considering a simplified model of psychotherapy, three diagnostic categories might be proposed. These are: the neurotic, psychotic, and character disordered. Table 1 below suggests the relationships between these categories, presenting problems and the possible efficiency of psychotherapy.

Table 1

Category	Possible Diagnosis	Effectiveness of Psychotherapy
Neurotic	Anxiety, depression, phobias	High
Character disorder	Criminal acts, drug addiction	Low
Psychotic	Schizophrenia, manic-depression	Low

As can be seen by the table, psychotherapy, in general, is most effective with essentially neurotic complaints and not very effective with character disorders or psychotic patients. There are, of course, many reports of successful treatment of these categories (Sloan, Stables, Cristol, Yorkton, and Whipple 1976) but it is important to note two considerations. First, there is a question as to whether the treatment of the character disorder or psychotic patient was successful because it dealt with a neurotic overlay which resulted from the difficulties encountered in the community and the elimination of these neurotic features accounted for the improvement. For instance, in a study of the therapeutic treatment of drug addicts (Zuckerman et al. 1975) it was concluded that the underlying character disorder was untouched while the neurotic overlay was dealt with. This could be the case in other studies demonstrating improvement in populations which could be designated as character disordered or psychotic.

A second consideration may be more to the point. The judgement of effectiveness depends on whether or not the problem can be fairly completely eradicated in almost every patient in the diagnostic group as opposed to whether their behavior can be managed for a short time. In sum, it depends on the generalizability and maintenance of the therapeutic operations (Bandura 1976). Relative to the psychotic patient, it appears psychotropic medication is the favored treatment at this time. Recent research is focusing on primary biological factors and initial results are quite encouraging. There are many successful instances of conditioning verbal behavior in schizophrenics and operant control of psychotic patients while they are on neuropsychiatric hospital wards (Ayllon and Azrin 1965; Schaefer and Martin 1966; Atthowe and Krasner 1968), but the large number of psychotic patients still hospitalized is eloquent testimony to the general effectiveness of any form of psychotherapy which proports to "cure" these patients. Similarly, the number of criminal offenders and drug addicts (National Institute of Law Enforcement and Criminal Justice 1977a) presently incarcerated also belies any attempt to assert that an effective method of psychotherapy for these populations has been fully developed.

This, of course, is not to imply that effective means of treatment may not be in the process of development at this time. There are a number of methods which have demonstrated potential (National Institute of Law Enforcement and Criminal Justice, 1977b) but as yet their promise has to be conclusively demonstrated.

Thus, it can be concluded that psychotherapy is most effective with neurotic patients. Indeed, success rated as high as 80% (Sloan et al. 1976; Wolpe 1958) are reported in the literature.

Treatment

Psychotherapeutic treatment is such a diverse area as to almost defy description. This section will, therefore, discuss three general considerations relative to the conduct of psychotherapeutic treatment. These are (1) various methods of interaction between therapists and patients, (2) focus of intervention of the therapist; and (3) essential elements of psychotherapeutic treatment.

Relative to the first of these, methods of interaction between therapist and patient, it is an often overlooked area of investigation which is presently receiving increased attention. Basically, methods of interaction are three types: face-to-face, media, and consultation.

Face-to-face interaction is the classic mode. In addition to the weight of tradition, it has the advantage of having been the subject of the majority of research investigations. The face-to-face situation provides the maximum flexibility and adaptability to the present situation, yet is most costly in terms of therapist time and expertise.

Psychotherapeutic treatment by the media is currently a major area of research interest. Media approaches can vary from the use of a computer for the administration of desensitization (Lang 1969) to bibliotherapy

(Horton and Johnson 1980) and videotape presentation (Hosford, Moss, and Morsell 1976) among others. In general, some fairly positive results have been forthcoming for the use of media approaches(Lang 1971).

Consultation also seems to be enjoying a great deal of current interest (Dinkmeyer and Carlson 1973). Generally, it has been characterized by a mental health professional teaching and aiding other professionals and paraprofessionals in the provision of psychotherapeutic services. Given research which suggests that the paraprofessionals can be effective counselors (Traux and Michael 1971) and behavioral engineers (Allyren and Michael 1959) and the increasing demands on professional time, it would appear that this trend is likely to flourish.

Therapist

The second area of consideration is the focus of intervention of the therapist. Essentially, the focus can be seen as three possible means. These are: individual psychotherapy, group psychotherapy, and institutional or community psychotherapeutic intervention. These foci correspond to the usual approaches by which a therapist attempts to treat a patient. For example, a therapist may wish to see the patient as an individual. This has an advantage in that the patient is the cynosure of the therapist's attention and that there are minimal impediments to immediately delving into any relevant aspect of the patient's past or present life situations.

Group psychotherapy and institutional psychotherapeutic intervention refer to situations where the therapist deals with a number of patients at the same time. Although the therapist loses a certain amount of adaptibility to the individual's functioning at the immediate moment, there are advantages. The therapist can enlist the cooperation of other persons for therapeutic purposes (Dinkmeyer and Muro 1971). The classic distinction between the foci is made on the simple variable of number of persons treated at one time. Since it is considered unethical for a psychotherapist to treat more than sixteen persons at one time (Shostron 1969), this is a convenient cutting point to differentiate group psychotherapy and institutional or community psychotherapeutic intervention.

CRITICAL ELEMENTS OF PSYCHOTHERAPY

The following is a discussion of the essential elements of psychotherapeutic treatment. This is a rather difficult task since controversy over the effective ingredients has been raging since the beginning of time. In perhaps the best controlled investigation of psychotherapy so far, Staples, Sloane, Whipple, Cristol, and Yorkston (1976) found that "successful treatment may be more of a function of the patient than any specific therapeutic procedures," (p. 349). Interestingly, in both short-term analytic psychotherapy and behavior therapy, the patient's speech patterns were predictive of improvement on outcome criteria (Staples et al. 1976). A further disturbing note is the review article by Kazdin and Wilcox (1976) which found "on purely methodological grounds, it appears that nonspecific treatment effects, at least at present, cannot be ruled out in accounting for the effectiveness of desensitization" (p. 724). Essentially, this suggests that nonspecific therapeutic effects such as treatment credibility, demand characteristics and expectancies for therapeutic change generated by treatment, could be the variables that actually cause the improvement seen by patients who undergo systematic desensitization. When one considers that in the Smith and Glass study (1977) systematic desensitization appeared far and away the most effective single psychotherapeutic treatment modality available at this time, the implications are shattering. In short, what appears to be rather persuasive evidence for the effectiveness of psychotherapy may truly be indistinguishable from placebo effects (Shapiro and Morris 1978). The obvious question arises, how do we know psychotherapy is effective? It would appear that while there is some doubt (Eysenek 1952, 1965), a number of reviews (Bergin and Lambert 1978; Smith and Glass 1977) have found evidence which found that psychotherapy is effective. While the most parsimonious conclusion would be to consider the evidence suggestive rather than conclusive, for the purposes of this book, the argument that psychotherapy is effective (at least with some patients) will be assumed. Unfortunately, there is not clear validation of any particular form of therapy (Smith and Glass 1977). Although the leaders appear to be cognitive-behaviorally oriented (systematic desensitization, rational emotive therapy, behavior modification) for some unexplained reason (Smith and Glass 1977), they seem to have missed this point through what appears to be some rather convoluted reasoning and unnecessary gymnastic data classification.

Since a search for the critical elements in psychotherapy through empirical research findings does not appear likely to be fruitful, at this time a conceptual analysis is suggested. While not the preferred method, it is the only avenue available given the lack of truly definitive literature reviews.

The relatively confused results of recent attempts to delineate the crucial effective elements in psychotherapy are instructive in that they suggest two different explanations. First, psychotherapy, as a whole, is relatively ineffective. For many reasons (pride, vanity, and wishful thinking among others) this is an unattractive alternative. Second, psychotherapy is a *very* complex process and our present mixed results are simply a reflection of this unkind truth. Clearly, the second is more preferable from both professional and scientific perspectives.

The burning question, however, resides with the amount of data one can marshall to support the second alternative. Happily, there appears an extremely solid basis upon which to rest an edifice of conjecture.

Generalizability theory (Cronbach, Glesner, Nanda, and Rajanatnon 1972) is a possible framework within the context of which to examine past results of psychotherapy research.

Generalizability Theory Applied to Psychotherapy

Although generalizability theory is rather complex, the essential elements can be briefly summarized. Simply put, generalizability theory is an application of the analysis of variance model to reliability theory. Classic reliability theory postulates each observed test score as two parts; these are true score and error. While this reasoning was straightforward, it neglected to explain differences in error terms found by different methods of computing reliability (split-half verses test-retest methods, for instance). Moreover, the elegant simplicity of classic reliability theory was obtained at the cost of including within the error a number of heterogeneous factors. In generalizability theory, many facets of possible variation are examined. These include components due to temporal variation of major interest, the true score. This more complex conceptualization of the variation which makes up any observed test score is taken from Fisher's factoral analysis of variance approach to experimental design. While at times maddeningly complex, it has the advantage of providing a very powerful and precise estimate of the true score and also the possible variation that an observed score will show when viewed in different situations.

Applied to psychotherapy research, generalizability theory has a potential value in elucidating the very complex processes which constitute psychotherapeutic intervention. Essentially, the three major variables we had delineated earlier, therapist, patient, and treatment are evaluated at the same time as all of these possible interactions (in the best of all possible cases). That is to say, there are separate variance components for therapist effects, treatment effects, patient effects, therapist-treatment effects, therapist-patient effects, treatment-patient effects, and therapist-treatment-patient effects. Basically, it is a classic fully crossed analysis of variance. Now it is instructive to observe the important points of difference between this design and the vast majority of research investigations of psychotherapy. In most studies, the cardinal focus is upon the treatment variable. That is, does treatment appear to cause an effect on outcome or process variables? Indeed, in almost any professional journal which reports psychotherapy studies, this is the most commonly printed study. The salient features are that therapist and subject effects are assumed negligable or controlled for by some sort of cross-over design feature. While this enables researchers to deal with a simplified situation, it also prevents what could be a more realistic representation of the manifold complexities of the actual psychotherapy situation. In the few studies which have at least approximated such a complex analysis of variance components modeling of psychotherapy (Howard, Orlinsky, and Perilstein 1976; Moos and Clemes 1967; Van der Vees 1965), it appears that, without going into great complexity, the major effect of treatment seemed to account for a relatively small percentage of the total variance while the majority of the variance was accounted for by interaction effects. In practical terms, this means global treatments do relatively little, but what is done during psychotherapy sessions, to whom and by whom, means a great deal. In other words, *interaction effects* seem to be the most fruitful area for future research inquiry.

Now, how does this compare with our previous discussion of traditional conceptualizations of psychotherapy research? Perhaps a diagram would be helpful. The traditional approach explores therapist effects, and patient effects as linear variables.

Traditional Conceptualizaton

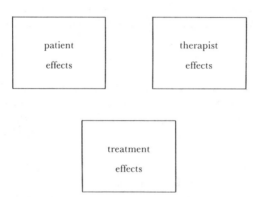

That is, ignoring the interactive nature of these variables in the psychotherapy process. A generalizable model would view the matter somewhat differently.

Generalizability Model Conceptualization

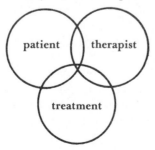

As can be seen in the generalizable model, all facets are crossed and the possible interactions are, at least assumed to be, possible. Statistical advantages aside, this model provides a possible explanation for the relatively low success of previous research efforts to identify the crucial elements in psychotherapy.

Simply put, it would appear that the majority of the variance to be accounted for in psychotherapy research is a function of emergent events in the particular session (Howard, Orlinsky, and Perilstein 1976). That is, who the therapist is and who the patient is, as we see them through the lenses of stable personality traits, are relatively poor predictors of outcome in psychotherapy. The essence of successful psychotherapy would appear to be interactional responding or, to put it another way, the care of the right therapist with the correct technique for the appropriate patient at the critical time. For example, it may be a client-centered therapist using systematic desensitization with a female neurotic's rose phobia, just the time when she ceased to receive secondary gain for being "sick," could be the optimal psychotherapeutic intervention for that particular patient, therapist, and treatment.

Future Decisions

Two possible directions of many in psychotherapy (Strupp 1978), with particular relevance to the aging, will be discussed. The first will deal with changes in the mental health system with regard to the elderly. The second direction will deal with a more general trend in psychotherapy, that is, toward multi-modal models.

Regarding changes in the mental health system, the overall thrust will be doing more with less money. The entire United States economy will be under financial pressure and the mental health system will not be spared. Gatz, Smyer, and Canton (1980) suggest that the intent to make efficient use of scarce money will bring community-based services, decentralization, increased planning and coordination, social-support systems, and targeting services to the most vulnerable, among other changes. While age doesn't guarantee wisdom, the elderly are, generally speaking, careful consumers. Quite likely, their collective influence on the mental health system will be in the direction of demands for increased accountablity and more cost-effective services.

At the present time, a trend towards greater eclecticism among psychotherapists appears to be strong and salient. No longer do behaviorists propose that rats are entirely adequate models for human behavior nor do psychoanalysts abhor short-term treatment. As others have said, psychoanalysis is "no longer deep in the heart of cathexis" and behavior therapy is not presently fully committed to the doctrine of the "immaculate perception."

A number of authors have remarked on movement toward fusions of existing therapeutic approaches (Garfield and Kutz 1976; Mahoney 1977; Goldfried and Davidson 1976; Lazarus 1976). Perhaps one of the most endearing anecdotes to emerge from this development was told by a behavior therapist concerning his practicum experience. He had received a rather strong radical behaviorist academic training and had just been placed in his first applied setting. During his first supervisory session, the staff psychologist, loking somewhat guilty and sheepish, took out a copy of Sullivan's *The Psychiatric Interview* and presented it to the trainee, with the comments, "this might be helpful to you when you begin seeing real people." So much for covert allegiance to the behavioral paradigm despite all odds.

As with any other complex conceptual phenomena, there are numerous and varied reasons for the present trend toward an amalgamation of therapy strategies. Two which may be of singular importance, refer to the power of therapeutic approaches and the general effectiveness of all therapeutic endeavor.

Regarding the first of these, the power of a therapeutic approach, there appears to be a universal consensus. That is, any form of therapy could stand an augmentation of clinical effectiveness. For example, consider the behavioral treatment of obesity. While numerous methodologically well-designed and skillfully executed studies have documented statistically significant results, the actual clinical utility of these findings leaves something to be desired. That is, behavioral treatment can help an overweight subject lose a few pounds fairly effectively   but no more than ten to fifteen with great intersubject variability (Jeffery, Wing and Stunkard 1978). So, while on one hand it should be noted at least statistical significance can be obtained, the search for a clinical effectiveness with all clients continues.

The second reason refers to the general effectiveness of all therapeutic endeavors. A recent meta-analysis of psychotherapy research (Smith and Glass 1977) found that the twelve major therapeutic approaches could each claim some clinical effectiveness. Although some theoretical schools appeared to have a larger effect size, none was without some demonstrations of positive change with human subjects. Even more surprising, a comparison between what many contemporary workers would consider the most firmly established approaches to therapy, psychoanalytically-oriented psychotherapy and behavior therapy, found a photo finish with behavior therapy ahead by a nose (Sloane, Staples, Cristol, Yorkston, and Whipple 1975), but roughly an 80% rate of patient improvement for a primary neurotic population. While it is possible to quibble about the outcome measures (assessor's ratings were based on patient interviews) and relative patient responsiveness (behavior therapy was more effective with more severely disturbed patients), in the end it must be concluded there are effective elements in both approaches even though each is very different in conceptualization, rationale for treatment, and actual methods.

Thus, it is becoming clear that no one therapeutic school of approach holds the ultimate answers. Yet, at the same time, it is also difficult to exclude any theoretical school or approach on the basis of demonstrated therapeutic impotence. Of course, part of the problem could be attributed to the article review policies of professional journals. As noted by Mahoney (1976), usually only significant results and innovative studies are selected for publication, thereby giving readers a somewhat distorted picture of rampant therapeutic success. But even allowing for this source of error, there appears to be two basic conclusions which can be drawn, as long as one accepts the premise that psychotherapy is effective. First, no one therapeutic approach has been demonstrated to have a total solution to actual clinical problems. Second, most therapeutic approaches can demonstrate, some, at least statistical, effectiveness.

Because of this situation, which some would regard as a certain maturing of the field of psychotherapy, the aforementioned trend to combine various therapeutic methods from, sometimes, very divergent approaches has emerged.

In conclusion, it might be noted that this chapter has attempted to introduce the reader to the psychotherapy of the aged. The characteristics of the elderly were delineated, an overview of the basic elements of psychotherapy provided and possible future directions outlined. The expectation, and hope, is that this chapter and the ones that follow will serve to help ameliorate the mental health problems of individuals of advanced years.

References

Atthowe, J. M & Krasner, L. A preliminary report on the application of contingent reinforcement procedures (token economy) on a "chronic" psychiatric ward. *Journal of Abnormal Psychology,* 1968, *73:* 37-43.

Ayllon, T. & Azrin, N. H. The measurement and reinforcement of behavior of psychotics. *Journal of the Experimental Analysis of Behavior,* 1965, *8:* 357-384.

Ayllon, T. & Michael, J. The psychiatric nurse as a behavioral engineer. *Journal of the Experimental Analysis of Behavior,* 1959, *2:* 323-334.

Ashly, J. D., Ford, D. H., Guerney, B. G., Jr., and Guerney, L. F. Effects on clients of a reflective and leading type of psychotherapy. *Psychological Monographs: General and Applied,* 1957, *71,* (24, whole No. 493): 1-32.

Baltes, P. B. & Labourie, G. V. Adult development of intellectual performance: Description, explanation, and modification. In C. Eisdorfer & M. P. Lawton (eds.), *The psychology of adult development and aging.* Washington, D.C.: American Psychological Association, 1973.

Bandura, A. Effecting change through participant modeling. In Krumboltz, J. D. & Thorenson, C. E. (eds.) *Counseling methods.* New York: Holt, Rinehart, and Winston, 1976.

Barak, A. & LaCrosse, M. B. Multidimensional perception of counselor behavior. *Journal of Counseling Psychology,* 1975, *22*: 471-476.

Bergin, A. E. & Lambert, M. J. The evaluation of therapeutic outcomes. In S. Garfield & A. Bergin (eds.) *Handbook of psychotherapy and behavior change: an empirical analysis,* (2nd Ed.), New York: Wiley, 1978.

Birren, J., Bick M., & Yiengst, M. The relation of structural changes of the eye and vitamin A to elevation of the light threshold in later life. *Journal of Experimental Psychology,* 1950, *40*: 260-66.

Butler, R. N., & Lewis, M. *Aging and mental health.* St. Louis, Mo.: Mosby, 1977.

Brody, J. Organization of the cerebral cortex: III—a study of aging in the human cerebral cortex. *Journal of Comparative Neurology,* 1955, *102:* 511-56.

Cronbach, L. J., Gleser, G. C., Nanda, H., & Rajaratham, N. *The dependability of behavioral measurements.* New York: Wiley, 1972.

Dinkmeyer, D. & Carlson, J. *Consulting: facilitating human potential and change processes.* Columbus, Ohio: Merrill, 1973.

Dinkmeyer, D. C. & Muro, J. J., *Group counseling: theory and practice.* Itasia, Illinois: E. E. Peacock Publishers, Ind., 1971.

Eysenck, H. J. The effects of psychotherapy: an evaluation. *Journal of Consulting Psychology,* 1952, *16*: 319-324.

Fiedler, F. E. A comparison of therapeutic relationship in Psychoanalytic, Nondirective, and Adlerian Therapy. *Journal of Consulting Psychology, 14:* 436-445.

Freud, S. On psychotherapy. In *Collected papers,* Vol. 1, pp. 249-263. London: Hogarth Press and the Institute of Psychoanalysis, 1950.

Garfield, S. L. Research on client variables in psychotherapy. In S. Garfield & A. Bergin (eds.), *Handbook of psychotherapy and behavior change: an empirical analysis,* (2nd Ed.). New York: Wiley, 1978.

Garfield, S. L. & Kurtz, R. Clinical psychologists in the 1970's. *American Psychologist,* 1976, *31*: 1-9.

Gatz, M. Smyer, M. A. & Lawton, M. P., The mental health system and the older adult. In L. Poon (ed.) *Aging in the 1980's.* Washington, D.C.: American Psychological Association, 1980.

Goldfield, M. R. & Davidson, G. C. *Clinical behavior therapy.* New York: Holt, Rinehart and Winston, 1976

Horn, P. Rx sex for senior citizens. *Psychology Today,* 1974, *8*(1): 18, 20.

Horton, A. M., Jr. Neuropsychological corelates of impaired brain functioning in the elderly: implications for behavior therapy. Paper presented at the Symposium: Behavioral assessment and treatment of elderly persons (Richard A. Hussian, Chair), 14th Annual Association for the Advancement of Behavior Therapy (AABT) Convention, New York City, November 21, 1980.

Horton, A. M., Jr. & Johnson, C. H. Rational emotive therapy and depression: clinical case study. *Perceptual and Motor Skills,* 1980, *51*: 853-854.

Hosford, R. E., Moss, C. S. & Morrell, G. The self-as-a-model technique: helping prison inmates change, In J. D. Krumboltz & C. E. Thorenson (eds.), *Counseling Methods.* New York: Holt, Rinehart, and Winston, 1970.

Howard, K. I., Orlinsky, & Perilstein, J. Contribution of therapists to patients' experiences in psychotherapy: a component of variance model for analyzing process data. *Journal of Consulting and Clinical Psychology,* 1976, *44*: 520-526.

Hurlock, E. B. *Developmental psychology.* New York: McGraw-Hill, 1968.

Jeffrey, R. W., Wing, R. R. & Stunkard, A. J. Behavioral treatment of obesity: the state of the art, 1976, *Behavior Therapy,* 1978, *9*: 189-199.

Kazdin, A. E. & Wilcoxon, L. A. Systematic desensitization and nonspecific treatment effects: a methodological evaluation. *Psychological Bulletin,* 1976, *83:* 729-758.

Kiesler, D. V., Some myths of psychotherapy research and the search for a paradigm, *Psychological Bulletin,* 1966, *65:* 110-136.

Kramer, M., Tauke, C. A. & Redick, R. W. Patterns of use of psychiatric facilities by the aged: past, present, and future. In C. Eisdorfer & M. P. Lawton (eds.), *The psychology of adult development and aging.* Washington, D.C.: American Psychological Association, 1973.

Kroger, W. S. & Fezler, W. D. *Hypnosis and behavior modification: imagery conditioning,* Philadelphia, F. J. Lippincott Co., 1976.

Lang, P. J. The application of psychophysical methods to the study of psychotherapy and behavior modification. In A. E. Bergin & S. L. Garfield (eds.), *Handbook of psychotherapy and behavior change: an empirical analysis. New York: Wiley, 1971.*

Lang, P. J. The on-line computer in behavior therapy research *American Psychologist, 1969, 24:* 236-239.

Lazarus, A. A. *Multimodal behavior therapy,* New York: Springer, 1976.

Luborsky, L., Singer, B., & Luborsky, L. Comparative studies of psychotherapies: is it true that everyone has one and all must have prizes? *Archives of General Psychiatry,* 1975, *32:* 995-1008.

Mahoney, M. J. Reflections on the cognitive-learning trend in psychotherapy. *American Psychologist,* 1977, *32,(1):* 5-19.

Mahoney, M. J. *Scientist as subject: the psychological imperative.* Cambridge, Mass.: Ballinger, 1976.

Meltzoff, J. & Kornreich, M. *Research in psychotherapy,* New York: Atherton Press, Inc., 1970.

Mischel, W. *Introduction to personality.* (2nd Ed.). New York: Holt, Rinehart, and Winston, 1976.

Mischel, W. On the future of personality measurement, *American Psychologist 1977,32:* 264-254.

Moos, R. H. & Clemes, S. R. Multivariate study of the patient-therapist system. *Journal of Consulting Psychology,* 1967, *31:* 119-130.

National Institute of Law Enforcement and Criminal Justice, *Drug program in correctional institutions,* U.S. Government Printing Office, 1977 (b).

National Institute of Law Enforcement and Criminal Justice, *The criminal investigation process: a dialogue on research findings,* U.S. Government Printing Office, 1977 (a).

Rogers, C. R. The necessary and sufficient conditions for therapeutic personality change. *Journal of Consulting Psychology,* 1957, *22:* 95-103.

Schofield, W., *Psychotherapy, the purchase of friendship.* Englewood Cliffs, New Jersey: Prentice-Hall, 1964.

Schulderman, E. & Subek, J. Effect of age on pain sensitivity. *Perceptual and Motor Skills,* 1961, *14:* 295-301.

Shapiro, A. K. & Morris, L. A. Placebo effects in medical and psychological therapies. In S. L. Garfield & A. E. Bergin (eds.) *Handbook of psychotherapy and behavior change: an empirical analysis,* (2nd Ed.) New York: Wiley, 1978.

Shostrom, E. L., Group therapy: let the buyer beware, *Psychology Today,* 1969, *2:* 36-40.

Sloane, R. B., Staples, F. R., Cristol, A. H., Yorkston, N. J., & Whipple, K. Patient characteristics of outcome in psychotherapy and behavior therapy, *Journal of Consulting and Clinical Psychology,* 1976, *44:* 330-339.

Smith, M. L. & Glass, G. V. Meta-analysis of psychotherapy outcome studies, *American Psychologist,* 1977, *32:* 752-760.

Staples, F. R., Sloane, R. B., Whipple, K., Cristol, A. H., & Yorkston, N. Process and outcome in psychotherapy and behavior therapy. *Journal of Consulting and Clinical Psychology,* 1976, *44:* 340-350.

Strupp, H. H. Psychotherapy research & practice: an overview.'' In S. Garfield & A. Bergin (eds.), *Handbook of psychotherapy and behavior change: an empirical analysis,* (2nd Ed.), New York: Wiley, 1978.

Traux, C. B. and Carkhuff, R. R. *Toward effective counseling and psychotherapy: training and practice.* Chicago: Aldine, 1967.

Traux, C. B. and & Mitchell, K. M. Research on certain therapist interpersonal skills in relation to process and outcome. In A. E. Bergin and S. L. Garfield, (eds.), *Handbook of psychotherapy and behavior change.* New York: Wiley, 1971.

U.S. Department of Commerce, Bureau of the Census. *Projections of the population of the United States, 1977-2050.* (Current Population Reports, Series P-25, No. 704). Washington, D.C.: U.S. Government Printing Office, 1977.

Van der Veen, F. Effects of the therapist and the patient on each other's therapeutic behavior. *Journal of Consulting Psychology,* 1965, *29:* 19-26.

Willis, S. L. & Balties. Intelligence in adulthood and aging: contemporary issues. In L. W. Poon (ed.) *Aging in the 1980's.* Washington, D.C.: American Psychological Association, 1980.

Wolpe, J. *Psychotherapy by reciprocal inhibition.* Stanford, Calif.: Stanford University Press, 1958.

Zimmer, M., Sola, S., Masterson, J., & Angelone, J. U. MMPI patterns in drug abusers before and after treatment in therapeutic communities. *Journal of Consulting and Clinical Psychology,* 1975, *43:* 286-296.

Zuckerman, M., Sola, S., Masterson, J., & Angelone, J. U. MMPI patterns in drug abusers before and after treatment in therapeutic communities. *Journal of Consulting and Clinical Psychology,* 1975, *43:* 286-296.

Part One
Time-Honored Psychotherapeutic Approaches

2

Individual Psychotherapy with the Elderly

Ronald J. Karpf

HISTORY

Sometimes the most time-honored approach is also the most innovative and effective. Such is the story of individual psychotherapy with the elderly. Beginning with its origin in psychoanalysis and Freud (1924a, 1924b), through the brief approaches of Goldfarb (1953, 1955, 1956), up to and including eclectic approaches (Brink 1979; Karpf, 1980a), individual psychotherapy with the elderly has proven itself despite therapeutic nihilism from those outside the field (Eysenck 1966).

The first pioneer in the field was Dr. Lillian J. Martin (1944; and deGrunchy 1930, 1938) who founded the San Francisco Old Age Counseling Center in 1929. Having done this after retiring from an active career, she continued as its director until her death at the age of ninety-two. Based on much of the positive thinking and inspirational literature of the time (Coue 1922), Dr. Martin's approach was quite directive and can be said to be a forerunner of many of the self control (Mahoney 1974) and cognitive techniques (Ellis 1970) so popular today. There is much in her method that is redolent of contemporary psychotherapeutic "homework assignments" of the behavior modifiers (Marks 1978) and the self-help philosophy of Recovery (Low 1950).

The first step of the Martin Method was to take a comprehensive history and mental status examination; a brief series of psychological tests were also given to aid in the understanding of the patient. Early memories were stressed; dreams were ignored. Dr. Martin believed it was very important to get a holistic picture of the elderly person. Assets, in addition to liabilities, were emphasized.

In an enthusiastic, but somewhat naive and superficial manner, the patient was given corrective slogans to practice. An illustration would be, "Have I tried to solve rather than to forget my problems." The patient was encouraged to practice this form of self-control and thought stopping at home. When in the office the client would often fill out charts and quasi-reinforcement schedules concerning daily activities, budgeting, recreation, and future goals. As important to this method as its technique was the in-spirational note of the caring therapists who worked with an age group that was entirely ignored at that time. Dr. Martin's stated effectiveness probably owes itself as much to a placebo effect (Shapiro and Morris 1978) as to the variations of technique. In addition, she claimed her approach to be more successful in a few brief sessions than psychoanalysis; yet there was no theoretical framework and no rationale. The Martin Method faded during the Great Depression and World War II and is rarely quoted today.

Almost all of the important advances in geriatric psychotherapy in the first half of our century were in the area of individual psychotherapy. Group, family, and behavioral interventions have all been developed as theoretical stepchildren of individual approaches in the last twenty-five years (Rechtschaffen 1959). The salient individual approach has been psychoanalysis. Contrary to most writing on the subject, Freud's original therapy cases were all short-term or mid-range in length (Small 1979). On-ly in his later, more pessimistic, years did Freud see the need for lengthen-ing the procedure. Thus, psychoanalysis, particularly the psychoanalysis of Freud's earlier years, is indisputably relevant to individual psychotherapy with the aged. Freud belived that to know the cause of a neurosis would lead promptly to its solution and resolution. His emphasis was upon a quick diagnosis of the psychodynamics involved and their undoing through active interpretation.

On the negative side of the ledger, however, are Freud's ageism and negative prognostic attitudes about the applicability of psychoanalysis at an advanced age. Freud offered three reasons for these difficulties (1924a, 1924b). The first involved the limitations of the aged ego. The founder of psychoanalysis believed that after middle age the resources available to the ego diminished, concordant with a diminishing of id and libido. In this regard, Freud felt that this lack of ego resources made the plasticity of the personality shrivel and the elasticity of the intellect rigid. In essence, the ag-ed were felt to be beyond the education of insight. As will be seen, the em-pirical literature does not bear these facts out. Modifications from classical technique have been successfully attempted by many later clinicians in the field.

The second objection of Freud rested on his assumption that a com-plete life review had to include a complete anamnesis, an uncovering of all childhood memories similar to the analysis of a twenty year old. This objection was that early childhood memories would be lost irretrievably, and with this loss would go the effectiveness of analysis. The advanced age makes for a building of repression, much as a pyramid adds stone, until repression is completed by death itself. Ignored in this argument is that, just as in dreams themes occur over and over, so in one's life history is there a reoccurrence of behavioral themes. This is the very essence of the psychoanalytic concept of repetition compulsion. In fact, many current writers view an abundant life history as making for a richer and fuller analysis (Butler 1963). It is unlikely that Freud would give credence to this contention if he were alive today. Most writers after Freud did not.

Lastly, Freud raised a value issue and ethical objection which is quite *au courant* and may be read in many disputations against psychoanalysis in the current literature. He said that the length of the procedure and the investment of time and money was not "worth the candle" because of the few years that the elderly analysand had left to live. On the one hand, this contraindication could imply a devaluation of old age. It could imply that mental health is not as important in old age as in the younger years. On the other hand, the contraindication could imply a valuation of the adaptational force of symptoms and pathology, an acceptance of older persons as they are rather than as they should be. Unless the elderly patient views a lengthy analysis as an adventure to be explored in and of itself, the economics of therapeutic investment will always be an issue. This last objection has led many later clinicians to shorten classical analysis (Grotjahn 1951; Karpf 1977, 1978).

Freud's pupils, perhaps acknowledging their teacher's own flexibility under the ravages of time, were far more optimistic about the indications of analytic therapy to the old. Part of the reason was that the procedure itself was undergoing modification. Concern about the length of treatment emerged as Freud's theoretical understanding of psychodynamics enlarged. Time was never a factor in the treatment of young, upper middle class Viennese patients. Still, Freud preferred brevity. In his treatment of the famous composer Gustav Mahler, only six sessions sufficed. (Jones 1957). Other patients were often treated in a similar manner, sometimes by advice and suggestion. *Studies on Hysteria* (Breuer and Freud 1895) is replete with astonishing details in the history of brief therapy. Fenichel (1954) recommended its reading to those interested in short-term treatment.

In 1941 the Chicago Institute of Psychoanalysis sponsored a national meeting titled "Council on Brief Psychotherapy." This was the first time that successful brief therapy was acknowledged as possible. World War II had brought with it a concern for the traumatic neuroses of battle (Kardiner 1941). Other disasters, such as the catastrophic fire at the Coconut Grove night club in Boston led to further refinements of technique for immediate and quick interventions in emergencies (Lindemann 1944). Lastly, the

Chicago team of Alexander and French (1946) created a furor by advocating a "corrective emotional experience" as an alternative to lengthy analysis. All subsequent attempts at theorizing about short-term psychotherapy have added little beyond the basic principles set down by these creative and illuminating collaborators. The exigencies of social need contributed to the explosion of articles in the field (cf. Small 1979), until at last the American Psychoanalytic Association sponsored a two-day workshop in 1977 on Special Problems in Brief Psychotherapy.

The above brief history of brief psychotherapy will be very appropriate when we turn to models and techniques for individual psychotherapy with the elderly, because as techniques of individual intervention with oldsters were being explored, so were modifications of Freud's classical technique. With the claim that "the age of the neurosis is more important than the age of the patient," Abraham (1946) set the first optimistic note regarding individual analytic treatment with old people. In his paper Abraham described the successful analysis of four neurotic patients over fifty years old. Earlier, Jelliffee (1925) had made the strikingly accurate statement that there is a difference between chronological age and functional age. This difference is currently acknowledged as a fact in the literature (Busse and Blazer 1980). Jelliffee was quite specific that only certain patients were appropriate for classical analysis.

While the former writers discussed their successes as "transference cures," Grotjahn (1940) emphasized the immediate gratifications that the psychotherapist should make with a patient. He anticipated more modern developments in the treatment of the aged. He also foresaw the distinction to be made between insight and supportive therapy (Alexander 1944). Supportive techniques were to be used with those having a weak ego.Guidance, reassurance, a protective role, and permissive attitudes rather than an atmosphere of deprivation, were all to be part of the armamentarium of the supportive therapist. The issue was essentially whether the aged or younger ego could control the release of impulse and drive flowing from the course of treatment. Two patients, ages sixty and sixty-six, were discussed in this context of supportive psychotherapy. Alexander did not use these patients' ages as variables, but instead stressed their weakened ego-integrative capacity. One of the patients was not seen because insight was contraindicated. The other was successfully treated.

The new concept of supportive treatment modified analysis and analytically-oriented psychotherapy, Meerloo (1953, 1955a, 1955b), Hollender (1952), Weinberg (1951) and Lawton (1952) all incorporated the new ideas. At about the same time, Goldfarb (1953a, 1953b, 1955a, 1955b, 1955c) introduced a unique manner of performing brief therapy. The modified techniques were based on more positive prognoses of long-term geriatric psychotherapy. The therapist should play a more active role and engage the patient face to face on a chair rather than on a couch. All agreed that limited goals should be agreed upon by both therapists and patient at the beginning of treatment. Resistance became a major issue. The newer psychoanalysts felt that the extensive life history of the elderly person made for less resistance. Id derivatives were closer to consciousness and easier to interpret. Under these circumstances the therapist must tread gingerly lest he or she interpret defenses too deeply and flood the patient's ego with libidinized material that could not be coped with. This was essentially the reason that Alexander had proposed supportive treatment. The newer analysts felt that focusing and analyzing current problems were sufficiently deep. Genetic material should not be unsettled.

At about the time Freudian analysts brightened their outlook toward the elderly, psychoanalytically-oriented psychotherapy was shortening the time of treatment. As mentioned, Alexander and French (1946) and other psychiatrists who were concentrating on emergency procedures were having a cogent effect on their colleagues. By the 1950's short-term psychotherapy was a new but established modality. So were supportive interventions.

It was in this atmosphere and period that Goldfarb (1953a, 1955b, 1955c) published. Working with severely impaired in-patients, Goldfarb believed that the natural dependency of older people could be harnessed so that the patient transfers feelings of power and omniscience to the therapist. In very brief interviews of five to fifteen minutes Goldfarb and his associates allowed the patient small favors and an eventual illusion of mastery over the surrogate-parent therapist. The patient is encouraged to feel in control of his or her gratifications and is permitted to enjoy a dependency relationship which cannot be achieved in normal adult interaction. Many have claimed that Goldfarb's work was truly a landmark in geriatric psychotherapy (Rechtschaffen 1959) because his technique was directed solely for the elderly and was not a modification of any previous work. This is correct. In addition, the brevity of his once-per-week sessions was economical of busy staff time. On the other hand, Goldfarb's population was limited to the severe end of the spectrum of psychopathology. All patients were only seen in nursing home settings. His technique is hardly applicable to outpatients or indicated for those who are mildly and more moderately disturbed. Goldfarb counters this criticism by advocating the continued use of institutional settings. His technique stands today as valid for certain individuals and certainly a turning point in gerontologic treatment.

The 1960's and 1970's showed a growing interest in geriatric psychotherapy and an explosion of articles in the field (Birren and Renner 1977). The *Journal of Geriatric Psychiatry* was founded exclusively to treat intervention issues. Other gerontologic journals devoted more time to treatment themes. Sparacino (1979) and Kahana (1979) offer excellent reviews of the literature coming out at this time.

Wolff (1963, 1970) had been quite active in the field. He was one of the first to use outcome measures and also treat a variety of disorders, from neurosis to schizophrenia. In addition, many of the cases studied were so-called "hopeless" patients. Wolff repeated the themes of Alexander and others by offering ego-supportive therapy. Instrumental to his approach was catharsis and raising self-esteem. One discovery made was that insight was contraindicated in most of his patients.Although his outcome measures were hazy, Wolff reported significant improvement in over half the population treated. Forty-one percent of his patients were discharged from the hospital.

Verwoerdt (1969, 1976) also focused on supportive therapy. His reasoning for abandoning an insight approach echoed Freud: "It may be easy to arrive at insight, but there may not be much opportunity to do anything with it." Verwoerdt's approach aims at achieving consolidation of life gains and consummating one's life work rather than exhuming old conflicts. Organic impairment, it is claimed, makes this more difficult.

Chronic, progressive brain syndrome, however, as a disorder, has often been used as a scapegoat for contraindications for individual psychotherapy. More recent writers (Brink 1979) have emphasized that individual psychotherapy can prevent as rapid a decline in such cases. Further, individual treatment is useful in training chronic brain disorder patients to behave more adaptively to the confines of their limitations. It was estimated by Brink that psychotherapy is effective in half of all cases diagnosed with dementia.

Strong advocacy positions have been taken by many in the field (Butler 1960; and Lewis 1977). Ageism was coined by these writers, as was life-review therapy. It is felt there that the elderly spontaneously review their lives. With the aid of a trained mental health professional, aged patients can be helped to a degree of wholeness by reminiscence. A conscious, deliberate effort is made by these therapists to make their patients actively participate in the life-review process: written or taped autobiographies, reunions, reconstructing family histories, examining photo albums and scrapbooks, and encouraging the patient to document verbally or in writing his or her life's work. The optimism of Butler and his colleagues is infectious but it strays far afield of what many would consider psychotherapy. It is more in the nature of environmental modification although it has been quite successful. Death and anxieties about this taboo subject are confronted. Revitalization of older peoples' experience and reduction of the routine of many lives takes place. In sum, nevertheless, this approach is rarely interpretive and can best be categorized with the many supportive techniques encountered above.

Pfeiffer (1971; and Busse 1973) and Weinberg (1975a, 1975b) echo themes that reverberate from the analysts of the 1940's. Greater activity on the part of the therapist is one. Symbolic giving is another, thus acting as a partial substitute object for what has been lost in reality. Empathy and special transference and countertransference problems are raised as issues. They will be discussed later in this chapter. It should be remembered, nevertheless, that the themes are old ones being examined under new light. Few of these writers have advocated Goldfarb's approach of encouraging dependency. Most have felt that greater independence should be reinforced from the start and on through termination.

MODEL

A proper model to represent individual psychotherapy with the elderly must incorporate its history. Just as the history of individual treatment approaches subsumes psychoanalysis and its modifications, the Martin method, and short-term therapeutic techniques, so must a model of individual treatment.

Such a model is offered in figure 1. It takes into account the diversity of psychopathology and the uniqueness of individual needs. There is a bipolar tension between supportive techniques and uncovering—or insight—techniques, as there also is one between long-term and short term therapy. Both are on a continuum and no qualitative demarcations would do justice to the strategies.

Time Factor

	Short-term	Long-term
Uncovering	Short-term Uncovering	Long-term Uncovering
or		
Supportive	Short-term Supportive	Long-term Supportive

Figure 1. A psychoanalytic model for individual psychotherapy with the elderly.

The Time Factor

The first conceptual confusion lies in differentiating psychoanalysis from analytically-oriented psychotherapy. Both are uncovering, or insight, forms of treatment, although there are supportive elements to both. The long-term nature of both of these forms of treatment stem from the fact that structural change of the ego-id-superego homeostasis is the goal. Structural change implies prevention of any further psychopathology. In psychoanalysis the goal is total re-structuring of the id-ego-superego homeostasis toward a more subliminated balance. Psychoanalytically-oriented psychotherapy, less ambitiously, attempts to resolve conflicts that are hindering behavioral and ego functioning. There is an attempt at cure in analytically-oriented therapy, but it is not as all-pervasive as in psychoanalysis proper.

Technical variations will be discussed later but for the present it should be stated that psychoanalysis is performed with the patient lying supine on a couch with the analyst out of view. Analytically-oriented therapy is conducted face to face. Psychoanalysis usually requires the patient to be seen four to five sessions per week, whereas analytically-oriented therapy usually requires the patient to be seen once or twice per week. Most of the literature on individual treatment with the aged makes reference to therapy and not to analysis proper (Ronch and Maizler 1977).

The models of long term analytically oriented therapy are always based on an uncovering—or insight—approach.Uncovering psychotherapy and analytically-oriented psychotherapy are used as synonomous terms in the present chapter. Long-term treatment implies that the patient is seen a minimum of one to three years. Anything less than this we will refer to as short-term therapy. Each session in long term treatment lasts between forty-five minutes and an hour. The time period is strictly adhered to after the initial interview. The rationale for this is to minimize counter-transference difficulties and to present limits and structure to the patient. If the therapist, for example, lengthens the session when he or she feels gratified, or shortens the session due to patient resistance, this communicates to the patient that therapy is not exclusively for his or her pathology, and creates a therapeutic misalliance based on the therapist's needs rather than the patient's. Brief or short-term therapy often varies from this stricture, as Goldfarb indicated by his five to fifteen minute interviews (Goldfarb 1955b).

The rationale for the long-term nature of much of uncovering therapy is based on the necessity of insight. Insight into conflict areas and insight into transference and resistance is a slow process because of the need for understanding the childhood origins of the psychopathological symptoms. This process is accomplished by what are termed genetic or vertical interpretations. Interpretations of behavior in the present are termed interpersonal or horizontal. Current thinking has it that horizontal interpretations can be as effective as vertical ones (Karpf 1978, 1980b), thus shortening the process of uncovering therapy. Usually both types of interventions, along with certain others, are necessary for effective insight and uncovering of intrapsychic conflict.

The other rationale for the long-term nature of analytically-oriented psychotherapy lies in the theory of personality development and psychopathology. Basically psychoanalysis is a psychology of inner conflict. It views the mind as the expression of conflicting forces (Kris 1950). Some of these conflicts are conscious, some beyond awareness, or unconscious. The process by which certain elements are barred from consciousness is termed repression. Repression must be analyzed for a successful treatment. As will be discussed, the concept of repression is particularly apropos in individual psychotherapy with elderly. The older one gets, often, the more difficult to lift repression and recapture childhood traumatic experiences. This was Freud's reason for his pessimism regarding analysis in later life. Disputes surrounding this issue were the cause for modifications in analytically-oriented therapy with older adults.

It is this difficulty in interpretation, and difficulty with analyzing repression, which creates the long-term nature of much of uncovering therapy. The patient must learn about himself or herself by working through various interpretations and turning these interpretations into insight. Only insight that is deep and changes the structural balance of ego-superego-id energies will result in a cure.

One concept of psychoanalysis that is particularly important for understanding the aged is narcissism (Freud 1914). This phase in the development of Freud's thought came when he attempted to apply the methods of psychoanalysis to understanding the psychoses. Until this point only the neuroses had a specific etiology. It lay in the conflict and struggle between the libido, which was directed toward preserving the species, and the ego, which is the origin of the self-preservative drive. For the psychoses, however, a different conflict was posited—that between libidinal energies vested in the self in opposition to libidinal energies vested in the representation of objects in the external world. Falling in love, pride in one's own children, and group and marital formation are all narcissistic, although in a mature way. At its core, the human personality retains a considerable part of childish self-centeredness. The capacity to love and identify with others is the healthy part of narcissism. Disturbances in this process because of traumatic experiences or poor object relations contribute to the severe forms of psychopathology, the narcissistic character disorders, borderline personalities, and the psychoses.

Recent years have shown advances in Freud's concept of narcissim and its application to many of the conditions of the elderly (Lazarus and Weinberg 1980). Kohut (1971) has been the major innovator in this area. He distinguished two forms of infantile narcissism that play a major role in the development of the adult. First is the grandiose type where the infant once felt omnipotent in symbiotic fusion with the mother. The second is the idealized type where the infant introjects the idealized portions of the parents and thus develops an ego ideal. Failure to achieve one's lifelong ambitions or live up to the ego-ideal leads to feelings of shame and disappointment. Inferiority feelings result from an imbalance between the narcissistic aspects of oneself, the ego, and the superego.

Contrary to Freud's belief that pathological narcissism is in the realm of psychotherapy of the psychoses, some (Goldberg 1973) believe that treatment of neuroses and character disorders should also consider narcissistic aspects of the personality.

With the aged, narcissistic psychopathology manifests itself as recurring depression or defensive grandiosity. This is one of the reasons that affective disorders and paranoia are so common in old age (Zung 1980). Elders are quite vulnerable in this area because object loss is so common and libido becomes cathected to the self as a compensation for psychological injury. Anger, rage, despair, and withdrawal are thus frequent normative crises in the aged. Already existing pathological character traits are exaggerated due to narcissistic injury. Coping with brain damage, the loss of a spouse, or retirement, are all biopsychosocial stressors precipitating a narcissistic injury to self-esteem. According to the above theory, working through mourning and grief becomes a major part of uncovering therapy, whether long- or short-term. Sensitivity to blows in self-esteem and ego strengthening measures are as important in long-term therapy of narcissistic disorders as developing insight.

Even supportive therapy that is long term must come to grips with narcissistic psychopathology. The therapist must be always available with empathy and sensitivity. Long-term, supportive therapy can serve as an object restitution in some older patients. Therapy may truly become interminable here, but not necessarily on a once a week basis. Once a month sessions, or even being always accessible to a telephone call, or if in an institution, to a drop-in office visit, are part and parcel of long-term supportive treatment. Allowing the patient to idealize the therapist replaces the lost idealized parental imago in supportive work. The imago should not be analyzed or interpreted. Punitive superego pressure can be altered in this manner by readjusting the ego idea. The therapist here becomes a new source of satisfaction and gratification. The therapist can maintain healthier life satisfaction in his or her patient right up until death, even in chronic progressive brain disease.

The indications for long-term treatment over short-term are usually patient-specific. One general rule of thumb is that a geriatric patient should never be placed in long-term therapy if a short-term approach will suffice. Theoretical debates concerning the nature of structural intrapsychic change should be avoided, with an eye always aimed on pragmatism. Symptom resolution is the goal in long-term therapy. Symptom removal is the focused goal of short-term therapy. Even long-term supportive therapy can aid in the resolution of conflicts, particularly the conflict over dependence versus independence. Allowing the patient to become dependent on the healer spontaneously resolves the conflict if the general atmosphere is one of unconditional positive regard (Parloff, Waskow and Wolfe 1978), warmth, and empathy.

The therapist must be more active, less neutral, and less objective in short-term therapy with the aged. One should not assume that diagnostic assessment of the patient's assets and liabilities is uncalled for here. Some might assume a stance that says that a long-term approach can always be substituted for short-term approach if the latter does not work out. Each approach, however, has different goals and a different rationale, and it is often complex to change an elderly patient's expectations about the length of treatment once they are established. A proper diagnostic assessment, in addition to indicating length, should also indicate whether uncovering or supportive therapy is indicated.

Another criterion for long-term treatment over short-term treatment is the patient's motivation for self-exploration and introspectiveness. Many patients view insight as a goal and challenge unto itself, and will not settle for brief approaches. Another important indication is whether a biopsychosocial stressor has precipitated the event. If the precipitating event, such as unresolved grief and the reemergence of childhood conflicts surrounding object permanence and loss can be identified, and if the patient is motivated for the challenge of self-scrutiny, then the adjustment reaction can be used fruitfully for exploring unresolved genetic conflicts in long-term therapy.

Chronic physical problems, such as primary degenerative dementia, call for long-term supportive therapy. Long-term techniques can also be a substitute for narcissistic injury and object loss by substituting dependency needs onto the therapist. This is the long-term equivalent of Goldfarb's (1955c) illusion of mastery technique in brief interventions, where he manipulates dependency needs as an aspect of the positive transference. In the long-term version, positive transference is manipulated so that the therapist is seen as an advocate, friend, ally, and protective parent. Clinical experience suggests that the chronic dependence on psychoactive drugs in some elderly individuals can be lessened with this intervention method.

The most important process in short-term uncovering or supportive therapy is diagnosis, diagnosis, and more diagnosis. There is too little time for nonactively waiting for conflicts to emerge or for a transference constellation and neurosis to surface. Diagnosis is not universally accepted as a prelude to treatment in long-term uncovering or supportive therapy, though it is emphasized as important in the present chapter.

There is a difference in diagnostic procedures between long-term and short-term techniques. In long-term treatment the pre-morbid personality is the focus of diagnosis. In short-term therapy nosology is not as important. Achieving a focus (Malan 1963, 1976) for the brief treatment is a major goal. Identifying the crisis situation and the current problem leads most quickly to the diagnostic formulation and, consequently, to the treatment.

In addition to an assessment of the crisis, an assessment of defenses, of ego functions, and of suicidal potential is crucial. The elderly are the most likely of all patients to carry out suicidal wishes and constant alertness to this fact is important. The affect of depression is not always paramount in suicidal danger. Impulsivity should be carefully reckoned with also. Frequent insomnia, weight and appetite loss, constipation, fatigue and diminished interest in sexual activity and hobbies all are important clues (Wolberg 1965). It is common knowledge among suicidologists that the twilight stages of depression, the initial onset and the onset of improvement are the times for the greatest caution. Rumination about suicide is more serious than transitory thoughts. A family history of suicide and structured plans on how the death wish will be carried out are prodromal signs. It is also important to know that suicide is highest after divorce and widowhood (Bunch 1972).

Therefore, an assessment of the crisis, its identification and explanation, and the biopsychosocial stressors involved are more important in assessment with short-term methods than the pre-crisis personality. The assessment of defenses and ego functions are important in determining whether negative transference interpretations can be effectively utilized by the patient. Ego readiness is thus an important criterion (Karpf 1980b).

Short-term therapy does not deal solely with emergencies, but it does aim at coping with crisis. A crisis is a possiblitiy for growth and further maturation. Regression to maladaptive reactions can take place if the therapist is not cautious. Further, the patient might resolve nothing and remain in a state of stress. There are, therefore, positive or negative possibilities. Short-term therapy with the elderly sets up specific goals in a brief time period to attack particular problems.

As stated previously, no aim is set for restructuring the personality or completely resolving conflicts, as would take place in long term approaches. The subjective relief of symptomatology is the aim. This usually occurs by catharsis or release of tension, mild ego strengthening, and lessening of superego pressure. Symptom-focused brief psychotherapy is, therefore, practical to institutions and ambulatory care settings. The emphasis is on limited goals, some understanding of the etiology of the difficulty, some recognition of current contributing factors, and some comprehension of measures that can remedy the difficulties. This form of treatment seeks modification of the incapacitating forms of psychopathology and the prevention of psychosis. It is often used in conjunction with pharmacotherapy. It should be the treatment of choice whenever the conditions do not look right for long term work. It is the indicated treatment for sometimes as simple a reason as lack of financial resources.

There are differences between short-term and long-term therapy in methodology. Small (1979) emphasized that all short-term therapists share one methodological dimension: "the concentrated focus of the therapeutic effort upon the symptoms or relevant matters only." The diagnostic process conceptualizes the problem. The therapist then chooses from a variety of intervention techniques to resolve the problem. In long-term uncovering therapy, relaxed listening, allowing the transference constellation to build, interpretation, and then working through of resistance and interpretation toward insight, are the chosen methods. There is no focus upon target symptoms and no time constraints. Some brief therapists, on the other hand, contract with their patients for a maximum of ten or twelve sessions. These clinicians feel that the limitation of sessions is motivating to the client and helps the focus of the therapeutic interaction. It also increases the need for activity and assertiveness on the therapist's part.

Uncovering or Supportive

Alexander (1944) set the original tone for differentiating uncovering from supportive therapy and his distinction still stands. His basic criterion was the strength of the ego. Uncovering treatment meant that the patient had to have the ego resources for insight, remembering, and working through. Supportive techniques were for everybody else. To this day supportive therapy is denigrated by viewing it as mindless hand-holding. Alexander viewed it as merely expedient. Only mild to moderate neuroses were indicated for uncovering therapy. The patient must be able to tolerate anxiety and be able to form a transference neurosis. Classical analysts today still feel that only neurotic transferences are appropriate in an analysis (Greenson 1967, 1972).

Since the 1950's, however, many more patients have been included in the widening scope for uncovering treatment (cf. Langs 1976). Pre-oedipal and pre-structuralized psychopathology were included in the more encompassing indications for uncovering therapy. Supportive treatment did not seem indicated as often as it had been in the past. Many now realize, however, that supportive therapy takes sound judgment and astute clinical skills (Herr and Weakland 1979). Proper training is necessary to carry out ego supportive treatment. If defenses are too weak or resistance too characterologically fixed in an older individual, it takes a knowledge of defense mechanisms and an understanding of resistance to realize this (A. Freud 1959).

Further, there are many supportive components to uncovering

therapy. After an interpretation, for example, the therapist must be gentle with defenses and supportive of any anxiety that is stirred up. Generally, however, supportive treatment is indicated in those older individuals who have deeply ingrained, characterological problems not amenable to insight. It is also indicated in most chronic progressive organic brain syndromes, including primary degenerative dementia arising in the senium. Long standing psychotic problems are most suitable for supportive work also. Certain reactive disorders involving the grief and loneliness of losing a spouse call for short-term supportive work. Any time the family of the aged person is brought into the session, and counseling techniques—i.e., advice and guidance—are used, supportive therapy is indicated.

The particular techniques of supportive therapy are advice, guidance, reassurance, assuming a protective role, permissive attitudes, and catharsis. The same need for proper training and experience is crucial in supportive work as in uncovering work. One cannot give sound advice unless it is based on knowledge of the disciplines of psychology, psychiatry, and gerontology, and also based on the ego function of sound judgment. Countertransference becomes, perhaps, more important an issue in supportive work than in insight work. This is because the therapists' mirroring function and neutrality are not adhered to. The therapist's personal biases, attitudes, and values become better known to the patient. Because there is more self-disclosure on the clinicians' side, there is more opportunity for inter-generational conflicts to come to the foreground. The therapist must be very careful not to impose attitudes or interests on the patient that were not there to begin with. Respect for the uniqueness and individuality of each patient is crucially important.

Uncovering therapy is analytically-oriented, yet not psychoanalysis itself. There is no need for five days a week on the couch when once or twice per week face-to-face in a chair will suffice. The only indication for psychoanalysis is the patient's desire for exploration and insight in and of itself. Not that analysis cannot be effective. As stated in the history section of this chapter, it already has proven to be so. Merely it is not necessary. Transference constellations resembling a transference neurosis can be elicited in analytically-oriented therapy.

Recent work has indicated (Langs 1976) that more primitive types of transferences are becoming more suitable for uncovering work. The new techniques are particularly helpful in hospital work with geriatric patients, a setting where psychopathology is likely to be more severe. Narcissistic, borderline and acute psychotic disorders present problems which are amenable to analytic work. These types of patients require parameters (Eissler 1953) to traditional work. Often a quest for infantile union becomes paramount in the relationship. The clinician must, therefore, guard against inducing regression in these patients. The transference conflicts in these non-neurotic patients often take on a personal flavor; hostility, extreme aggression, or seductive-like behavior may become prominent in the transference. Here is where neutrality and a firm grip on one's own maturity and ego strength become important. The therapist must respond with patience and consistency. Interpretations are the leverage that the clinician has at his or her disposal.

One aspect of commonality between uncovering and supportive therapy is the realm of nonverbal intervention (Karpf 1980b). Until recently, analytic investigations of therapy viewed transference manifestations primarily in terms of the patient's verbal communications. The only alternative to verbal discussion of fantasies was acting out of one's conflicts. Beginning with Winnicott (1965) and Balint (1968), however, a more holistic conception of the clinician's armamentarium was introduced. Global descriptions of certain nonverbal aspects of the therapist's stance alluded to the establishment and maintenance of the ground rules and boundaries of the therapeutic relationship, his or her concern for the patient, consistency, regularity of sessions, qualities of the silences, and the timing and tone of interpretations. All of these constitute an effort to create a special therapeutic atmosphere that offers the older patient a sense of security, safety, and an opportunity for catharsis. The elderly are often quite sensitive to what is left unsaid, the area of the nonverbal. The therapist must be prepared to sensitively respond to nonverbalized responses as well as verbal associations.

BASIC CONCEPTS

The basic concepts which are sound for individual psychotherapy with the aged are sound for individual psychotherapy throughout the entire life cycle.

All psychotherapy centers around the therapeutic relationship. The quality and nature of the relationship can enhance or severely impair effective therapeutic intervention. The *therapeutic alliance* involves the conscious, rational, and nonneurotic aspects of the relationship between patient and clinician. It is based on the patient's desire for improvement and maturation, and the healer's desire for effective treatment. An effective alliance ideally occurs between the responsible part of the patient's ego and the therapist's ego. Throughout treatment this alliance will weather many storms of neurotic and pre-oedipal anxieties and hostilities. It will allow the therapist to make specific interventions even though considerable dysphoric affect will be aroused. And it will sustain the patient's capacity to accept and integrate these interventions. Sustaining the therapeutic alliance takes considerable skills in supportive measures, skills which were discussed earlier.

Transference refers to the process of experiencing in the present, feelings and attitudes that originated in the past. With young and middle aged adults these fantasies, affects, and attitudes were originally experienced with earliest relationships, such as the parents. With the elderly, however, transference may occur that was originaly experienced with children or other extra-familial figures, such as teachers or doctors. Transference feelings can be neurotic, borderline psychotic, narcissistic, or psychotic, depending on the severity of psychopathology. The degree to which the elderly patient can distinguish the reality or nontransference section of the relationship from the fantasy or transference sections of the relationship, the stronger will be the therapeutic alliance and the more insight and less supportive work can be accomplished. The male clinician should be as non-chalant toward being the receptacle of erotic feelings from a beautiful twenty year old woman as from a charming seventy year old woman, although the latter is usually experienced by the clinician as disconcerting. When transference feelings crystallize around the therapist and the patient is neurotic, a *transference neurosis* is said to have formed. Nevertheless, borderline, narcissistic, and psychotic patients can form intense transference constellations centering around their particular pathology. A transference constellation occurs in uncovering treatment, but it is unlikely and actively discouraged in supportive therapy.

Countertransference refers to the therapist's transference reactions to the older patient. Countertransference is always inappropriate and arises from unconscious, unresolved conflicts in the therapist. It usually clouds his or her understanding and responsiveness unless self-analyzed. Some claim that countertransference can be used in the service of treatment, if it is a vehicle for better understanding of the patient (Sandler 1976). Due to lack of insight into the pathology, the patient will sometimes try to evoke certain roles and behaviors in the therapist which the patient finds gratifying. These must be openly analyzed and never acted upon by the therapist.

Regression, another feature of psychotherapy with the elderly, is the tendency of a patient to return to earlier, more childish and infantile patterns of thinking, feeling, and functioning. There are therapeutic and pathological aspects to regression. Normal regression in the service of the ego is adaptive and may be observed in adults during play and creative activity. During stress of any sort regression often becomes prominent. This is particularly true in the stress of physical illness and pain, conditions so common in later life. Therefore, much of the regression in older individuals is due to real precipitating events and cannot be attributed to the aging process itself.

Regression may be constructive in therapy if the therapeutic alliance is maintained and the patient continues to distinguish fantasy from reality. It must be a controlled regression induced by the therapeutic atmosphere and setting. When regression appears too rapidly or is too intense or too prolonged, it has a destructive influence on therapy. A complete diagnostic assessment must include the patient's capacity to tolerate therapeutic regression. When regression is already a significant part of the clinical picture it is undesirable to encourage it further. Regression to the level of earlier primary relationships allows the patient to form new object relationships if the patient's problems are pre-oedipal and pre-structural, and work through insights into the nature of these relationships if the conflicts are oedipal.

Resistance comprises all those elements and forces within the older patient, both conscious and unconscious, that oppose the treatment process. It is not surprising that a patient might oppose parts of treatment. The aim of therapy is either to restore a former psychological equilibrium or reestablish a new one. To reestablish a new equilibrium defenses must be interpreted and the anxiety and depression which were defended against must come to the foreground. The mobilization of resistance diminishes anxiety and restores the prior psychological homeostasis.

Other factors are also at work in resistance. Because the therapist provokes this disequilibrium the patient unconsciously blames the therapeutic process and the therapist for the anxiety and depression he or she suffers. Consequently defense mechanisms are mobilized to resist or oppose the therapy.

A dilemma now faces the therapist. In supportive treatment with the elderly, resistances are often allowed to remain intact. In uncovering therapy with older people on the other hand, resistance and defenses must be interpreted for treatment to progress. If the therapist attempts to reduce the resistances by bringing them into awareness, this effort may arouse extreme anxiety and induce further regression. If this happens the therapist must reverse his or her course and leave the current ego-supergo-id homeostasis intact. The chief diagnostic question here is how much anxiety can be tolerated without being overwhelming, and how much regression can be allowed without causing further pathology to emerge. In addition, the therapeutic alliance must be monitored for signs of a breach. If a misalliance occurs this must be corrected before any interpretive work can continue. *Transference resistance* is the most powerful form of resistance and the most difficult to work with. In this form of resistance positive or negative feelings are displaced from figures in the past onto the therapist and obstructs therapeutic progress by undermining the therapeutic alliance. The working through and resolution of such a resistance is crucial for therapy to progress and ultimately succeed.

Free association is the primary requirement of the patient in uncovering and even supportive long-term therapy with the elderly. Free association means that the patient must express all of his thoughts freely and openly, to say all that comes to mind without selectiveness, and regardless of whether the thoughts are embarassing or appropriate. Free association requires a split in the patient's ego functioning similar to the split necessary for the therapeutic alliance. Part of the patient's mind is allowed to drift into the unconscious and verbalize the thoughts that became conscious, and part of the patient must maintain a critical stance that analyzes these id derivatives. The therapist listens with meaningful and constructive empathy. He or she listens for the surface or manifest content in addition to the underlying or latent content. At all stages in treatment the therapeutic alliance must be monitored for breaches. Lack of empathy or excessive passivity on the therapist's part may cause a misalliance to occur.

Questions are one of the most significant parts of the therapist's armamentarium. Although most clinicians view questions as a means of obtaining information, the question can be a probing way of exploring the unconscious, or it can be a way of focusing the patient's attention on a specific issue. The therapist's sensitivity and empathy are salient points to consider in using questions. Usually open-ended questions or rhetorical questions, rather than those that require only a "yes" or "no" should be utilized. Clarification of ambiguity may be another reason for using questions.

Clarification may be used by repeating something the patient has said or done as a way of promoting further consideration of an issue or elaborating upon associations. Thus clarification can be confrontative or interpretive. It usually prepares the patient for an interpretation by bringing conflicts to the preconscious level.

Confrontation is a particular intervention which forcefully directs the patient's attention to conflicts or themes which are being avoided or denied. When used tactfully a confrontation can make the unconscious preconscious or the preconscious conscious by dealing with real situations or events in the patient's life. A solid therapeutic alliance must be had for confrontations to be effective, for sometimes a confrontation can be anxiety-producing and painful.

Interpretations are generally acknowledged to be the most important form of intervention in uncovering therapy. They are rarely used in supportive treatment. The interpretation is the deepest form of verbal intervention. It brings into conscious awareness and illuminates an area of conflict that was previously unconscious and repressed. Interpretations can be either horizontal or vertical. A vertical interpretation is genetic and developmental. It relates past experience to present feelings. Horizontal interpretations are interpersonal and dynamic in that they relate or connect feelings and defenses in the therapy office to those outside the office in everyday life.

Interpretations are the chief way to achieve insight and understand defenses and resistance. They must be used gingerly so as not to engage in "wild analysis." It is a common mistake for neophytes to interpret unconscious content too deeply for the patient's ego to cope with. The patient must be prepared via questions, clarification, confrontation, and more superficial interpretation, otherwise the therapist's interpretation can cause undue anxiety and subsequent pathological regression. Therefore, tact, timing and dosage or amount, are important factors in utilizing interpretation. Erroneous interpretations often reflect the therapist's inadequate understanding of the patient's material and could be a signal of counter-transference.

Working through, which begins after interpretation, is a laborious process for the patient because the insight and all of its ramifications must be explored, extended, and tested. Reconstructions of earlier life experiences may be helpful. They correlate and tie together all of the interpretations which had gone before. The patient learns to accept, integrate, and understand the basis of his or her psychopathology. At least a different psychological equilibrium has been established and the personality can be said to be partially reconstructed. Behavioral change will have taken place also.

BASIC CONCEPTS APPLIED

Transference is sometimes used in a different sense with geriatric patients than has been described here. The idea of "reversed transference" has been popular (Grotjahn 1955). In a reverse transference, the patient sees in the therapist a younger person. Instead of the usual oedipal relationship of father to son or mother to daughter, the patient becomes the parent and transference fantasies are directed to the therapist as child or grandchild. What will be analyzed in the therapy, therefore, is the oedipus complex in reverse. This is particularly true when the therapist is the same age as the child or grandchild of the patient.

No new concepts need to be understood with the "reverse oedipus complex." Taking the idea of regression to be central in uncovering therapy, and the idea of transference as an inappropriate displacement of past feelings onto the present, the clinician is thus made aware of the concept of *cumulative repression.* Cumulative repression refers to the accumulation and layering of memories throughout life, much as Khan (1963) has spoken of cumulative trauma throughout childhood and adolesence.

Repression of these various memories make some of the more recent memories more accessible to consciousness than others. Thus it is often not necessary to make genetic interpretations, relating childhood to adulthood. Instead, the process of remembering and working through can be accomplished by remembering aspects of the personality in young adulthood or middle age, and relating these to the present. This is what is meant by filial or parental transference, the reverse oedipal triangle. It is the partial regression and lifting of repression to an earlier stage of adult life, but not necessarily to childhood.

Two other forms of transference reactions are common with elders, the idealized transference and negative transference reactions. The idealized transference stems from infantile wishes to incorporate the omnipotent parent. Overidealizing the clinician can indicate that the patient despairs about himself or herself, or that he or she is projecting part of a grandiosity onto the healer. This transference reaction can be used supportively or interpretively, depending on the type of treatment. Maintaining the positive aspects of this kind of transference can be very supportive in feeling trust and security in the therapeutic alliance. It can also be uncovered by interpreting the feelings as similar to the patient's child to the parent, bypassing a vertical interpretation to childhood.

Negative transference reactions are quite common, sometimes for reasons founded in reality. General systems theory has postulated that sometimes a patient can be scapegoated and identified by others as the patient, whereas in reality, the system doing the labeling is pathological, a projection of pathology, if you will (Haley 1976). Under these circumstances a son may wish to gain hold of the family finances or a daughter may be denying marital problems. It would, therefore, be good reality testing and astute judgment to be angry, hostile, and bitter. More transferentially, sometimes the elderly patient feels humiliated by seeing a therapist or being put in a hospital. The patient may not understand the situation or fear that the therapist will not understand him or her. Accepting and tolerating the anger can produce a deep lasting trust for long-term therapy. The anger of the paranoid patient or the schizo-affective disorder usually comes from past disappointments with significant others.

Countertransference reactions of the negative variety are more common in working with older patients than with younger patients. The denial of the erotic and sexual nature of most elderly patients is the most common countertransference problem. Both Meerloo (1955b) and Grotjahn (1955) have noted the anxiety that is often engendered in younger psychotherapists. This attitude produces shame and confusion in elderly patients, thus compounding the pathological picture. Depression and guilt are frequent affects in widows who have lost spouses yet still desire the warmth and closeness that sexual contact brings. The denial of sexuality in the elder may be due to ignorance on the clinician's part or simply a misguided wish for the sanctity and sexual purity of old age.

The second common countertransference problem lies in what Meerloo (1955b) terms the narcissistic injury to the therapist's professional ego in many cases of irreversible decline leading eventually to death. The medical model upon which psychodynamic therapy is based is not a rehabilitation model with occasionally limited goals. It is a model for total cure. When this does not occur it wounds professional pride and may result in angry countertransference feelings.

The last countertransference problem singular to work with the aged lies in the relationship the therapist had with his own parents, and, perhaps, even grandparents. Unresolved oedipal conflicts and issues surrounding nurturance and dependency often are induced by older clients. Hostility toward parents frequently gets projected onto the oldsters, with the underlying fear being the unconscious identification with the patient's helplessness. A reaction formation to the anxiety aroused by working with the aged often lies in using superficial interpretations rather than deep ones, supportive therapy rather than uncovering therapy, and brief approaches rather than long-term ones. Watering down the therapeutic process may help the therapist suppress his or her hostility or any other dysphoric affect engendered by treatment.

Resistance in individual geriatric psychotherapy might stem from generational and socio-cultural differences, including education. Seeing a psychotherapist and committing oneself to the therapeutic endeavor could be resisted due to sheer ignorance of what is involved. The difficulty of treatment is thus increased. On the other hand, resistance, viewed intrapsychically as defense mechanisms, is usually more accessible to interpretation because it is less repressed, due to diminished ego control.

The memories that come to consciousness when resistance is analyzed in the aged are usually in the form of reminiscence. Reminiscences are a suitable substitute for reconstructions of the past. They can be interpreted genetically, or vertically, in that relating a young adult memory to the current circumstance of a seventy-five year old patient is the age-equivalent in interpreting a childhood memory to a twenty year old. What must be remembered is that repression is cumulative throughout life. Uncovering can reconstruct the development of adult life as effectively as childhood memories, usually with as much effectiveness.

Reminiscence has many other therapeutic functions. Butler (1963) has postulated that it is central to the life review process. It can cause a resurfacing of old conflicts and bring past transgressions and guilt to the conscious ego. Depression, therefore, is sometimes the result of the process of reminiscence. Nevertheless, this mental mechanism, by bringing conflicts to the surface, is a source of renewal. The evolution of candor, serenity and wisdom can be the by-products of reminiscence. If properly analyzed by the therapist, reminiscence can bring that lasting sense of self-esteem which Erikson (1963) has characterized as ego-integrity. Pincus (1977) maintains that, in addition to maintaining self-esteem, reminiscence reinforces a sense of identity by reinforcing a sense of wholeness and continuity to life as it has been lived.

The last intrapersonal function served by reminiscence is that it helps allay the anxiety associated with decline and death. The approach of dissolution and death, and the ability to see through one's childhood fantasies of invulnerability are interwoven. Themes of demise often pervade the dreams of older people. Reminiscence is often a healthy response to the biological and psychological fact of death.

In summary, therefore, reminiscence is not the meaningless babble of a deteriorated elder recalling the past, but a positive adaptational response to be encouraged by the therapist. The curiosity that non-depressed patients reminisce more than depressed ones makes reminiscence a possible outcome measure of successful psychotherapy.

The technical handling of reminiscence is not more complicated than other interventions. Reminiscence is the basic material and content of free association. The proper attitude of relaxed listening for elements of transference or resistance must be adhered to. Relating past to present should be handled in the same manner as an interpretation given to an adolescent or young adult. Timing, tact, and dosage of interventions into the content of the reminiscence must be based on the readiness of the aged ego for the interpretation.

CASE ILLUSTRATION OF SHORT TERM UNCOVERING THERAPY

Mr. K was a seventy-one year old white male who was referred by the social worker of a day care center. He was reported to be very anxious and to be having difficulty completing the activities in his program.

The patient's history showed him to be the youngest of six children. Father was described as a good man, but harsh and distant. Mother was described as similarly harsh and distant. Mr. K's school history was unnoteworthy, except that one of his brothers died of pneumonia during the elementary school years. He is a high school graduate with one year of business college.

The patient once received treatment at the age of eighteen from a psychiatrist. His mother had referred him at the advice of their family physician due to withdrawn and agitated behavior. Mr. K saw the psychiatrist for only a few weeks. His father died when he was twenty and his mother when he was twenty-seven. At thirty he married and later had two sons. Finally, after twenty-five years of marriage Mr. K's wife deserted him because she said that she could no longer cope with his problems.

Since then his work history has been unstable. He lost jobs because he could not concentrate and complete the work. The patient had lived in a boarding home for the last five years. At the Senior Citizens Day Care Center Mr. K participated in volunteer work and recreational activities twice weekly.

At the initial interview the patient was capable of forming rapport and, seemingly, a therapeutic alliance. The repesenting problems were obsessive ruminations about the failures in his life, such as his role as husband, father, and employee. These ruminations prevented him from concentrating on whatever activity in which he was engaged. Anxiety of a diffuse, free-floating type was prominent also.

The beginning stages of therapy set the symptomatic goals of treatment: first, to reduce his anxiety level; secondly, to reduce his obsessive ruminations. We decided to set a time limit of three months on the treatment and to renegotiate the contract if necessary. This limit was a necessary motivation for the patient.

Together we parceled out the precipitating factors of Mr. K's current crisis: one was a new roommmate at his boarding home and, two was the idea of moving to a new, more comfortable boarding home, initiated by his social worker. Finding the reality precipitates of his symptoms partially alleviated them during the first three sessions.

The middle segment of the treatment dealt with transference issues. His abrasive style of interaction with me was interpreted as contributing to his difficulty with his roommate. This was a horizontal interpretation. A vertical, or genetic, interpretation was offered in which I related Mr. K's inability to confront his social worker with his real wishes, to his passive feminine identification and relationship to his mother. All interpretations had to be repeated a number of times in various verbal styles and in different situations, in order for Mr. K finally to understand them and work them through.

Throughout the first and second months, Mr. K's obsessive ruminations about his "failures" in life became evident. The patient had introjected from his parents a harsh superego. This was clarified for him. We discussed a few situations from his adolescent and young adult years where the patient's identification with his parents' guilt made it difficult for Mr. K to fully enjoy any activities. At times the guilt and depression became very severe. The interpretations and clarifications helped alleviate the severity of the psychopathology.

Often it was necessary to point out the reality of Mr. K's past marriage. He blamed the divorce on himself rather than understanding that his wife shouldered much of the responsibility. Occasionally it was necessary to interpret how his relationship with his wife repeated Mr. K's relationship with his mother. Discussing the positive and negative elements of the marriage helped create a more holistic concept and helped integrate much of the object splitting that was taking place.

The terminal phase of treatment, the last three interviews, included a discussion of his transference feelings toward me. They were surprisingly strong in light of the brevity of our interaction. There was a sadness present but also a deep sense of gratitude. We adhered to our three month contract, nevertheless. We reviewed the gains made. He related better to his roommate and decided not to leave his boarding house. His anxiety and ruminations were considerably diminished. In addition, he resumed his recreational and volunteer activities in the day care center. Guilt and depression, though still present, were markedly diminished. I made it clear that Mr. K could return to out-patient treatment with me any time in the future if he or his social worker felt it necessary.

CASE ILLUSTRATION OF LONG-TERM SUPPORTIVE THERAPY

Mrs. C, a sixty-six year old black female, was admitted to a geriatric treatment center on an involuntary court commitment. Her neighbor had complained to the police about her bizarre behavior in the community. The court psychiatrist described her behavior as "euphoric, hyperactive, with grandiosity and a flight of ideas."

Mrs. C had a history of short-term hospitalizations during the preceding twenty years. She had been able to remain out of the hospital for four years before her symptoms began. Previous diagnoses were manic-depressive psychosis and schizo-affective disorder. Mrs. C had one son from a husband who had died three years ago. She rarely saw her child. Psychological testing was done and confirmed the court psychiatrist's impressions. Her diagnosis was schizo-affective disorder. After one month of observation, chemotherapy, and individual and group therapy, not enough improvement was evidenced for her to return to the community. She was transfered from the acute care building to the long-term care building.

It was then that I took the case. I realized that an insight approach was contraindicated and that Mrs. C's treatment should be long-term, in view of her psychopathology and the failure of a short-term approach.

The beginning phase of treatment centered on the therapeutic contract. It was necessary to build rapport and trust, but not necessarily a therapeutic alliance. Mrs. C was not going to have to observe herself objectively and achieve insight. I revealed some material about myself to the patient, concerning whether I was married, the ages of my children, and my training and educational background. This helped establish rapport. It was important to discuss her feelings about being treated by a young, white male. These difficulties were analyzed and led to a more secure and trusting relationship.

The ground rules of therapy were explained. We met twice weekly in the visitors' lounge. Also explained to the patient was the need for honesty and the requirement for discussing anything that comes to mind, no matter how embarrassing. By educating Mrs. C about the framework of our relationship I was orienting her to time (our therapy sessions), place (the waiting room) and person (me). Much of her dependency needs were quickly transferred to me.

Therapy did not have a clearcut middle and end. Catharsis and ventilation were prominent throughout. Talking to a supportive therapist in a secure setting was very reassuring. Interpretations were rarely used. Questions and clarifications were the chief analytic interventions. Through questions I made her aware of issues she was facing, such as could she eventually go to a nursing home, and could she control her emotions and occasional hyperaggression? We clarified her feelings. Usually she denied any awareness of anger or resentment at others. By reacting to the content of her sessions with the underlying feeling tone, Mrs. C became more aware of her affective life.

Denial was a prominent defensive maneuver. She could never discuss the death of her husband, which was three years previous to the present hospitalization. The patient could only tolerate a discussion of dying and death in an intellectualized manner. This apparently helped, nonetheless. Thus I accepted much of her defensive cognitive style so as not to raise too much tension. Session after session became anxiety suppressive. An interpretation would have raised intolerable anxiety and damaged the therapeutic relationship.

Advice and other counseling techniques were often part of the sessions. Mrs. C enjoyed my role as mental health expert and took a parent's pride that her doctor was so wise for such tender years. This positive transference was crucial to our work together because it gave my interventions an imprimatur that they might not have had for such a disturbed person.

Most of the treatment remained the same as months ran into two years. It was never boring, however. She had every staff member analyzed and her observations of everyone were often quite astute. Her interactions with other patients on the unit or current events in the news were frequent topics of the interviews.

Gradually her affective life stabilized and reality testing increased. Her euphoria and manic-like behavior were under control. At a team conference we decided that Mrs. C was appropriate for a nursing home placement. Her dependency needs made independent living an impossibility.

The patient was at first reluctant to go but changed her mind. After two years of treatment she left. A follow-up six months later found her to be doing well with only residual symptoms of her pathology.

References

Abraham, K. The applicability of psycho-analytic treatment to patients at an advanced age. In *Selected papers of psychoanalysis.* London: Hogarth Press, 1949.

Alexander, F. The indications for psychoanalytic therapy. *Bulletin of the New York Academy of Medicine,* 1944, *22:* 319-334.

Alexander, F. and French, F. *Psychoanalytic therapy.* New York: Ronald Press, 1946.

Balint, M. *The basic fault: therapeutic aspects of regression.* London: Tavistock, 1968

Birren, J. and Renner, V. J. Research on the psychology of aging. In Binen, J. and Schaie, K. W. (eds.) *Handbook of the psychology of aging.* New York: Van Nostrand Reinhold, 1977.

Breuer, J. and Freud, S. *Studies on hysteria.* New York: Basic Books, 1895/1957.

Brink, F. L. *Geriatric psychotherapy.* New York: Human Sciences Press, 1979.

Bunch, J. Recent bereavement and suicide. *Journal of Psychosomatic Research,* 1972, *163:* 361-372

Busse, E. and Blazer, D. The theories and processes of aging. In Busse, E., and Blazer, D. (eds.). *Handbook of geriatric psychiatry.* New York: Van Nostrand Reinhold, 1980.

Butler, R. Intensive psychotherapy for the hospitalized aged. *Geriatrics,* 1960, *15:* 644-653.

Butler, R. The life review: an interpretation of reminiscence in the aged. *Psychiatry,* 1963, *26:* 65-76.

Butler, R. and Lewis, M. *Aging and mental health: positive psychosocial approaches.* St. Louis: Mosby, 1977.

Coue, E. *The practice of autosuggestion.* New York: Doubleday, 1922.

Eissler, K. The effect of the structure of the ego on psychoanalytic technique. *Journal of the American Psychoanalytic Association,* 1953, *1:* 104-143.

Ellis, A. *The essence of rational psychotherapy: a comprehensive approach to treatment.* New York: Institute for Rational Living, 1970.

Erikson, E. *Childhood and society.* New York: W. W. Norton, 1963.

Eysenck, H. J. *The effects of psychotherapy.* New York: International Science Press, 1966.

Fenichel, O. Brief psychotherapy. In Fenichel, H. and Rapaport, D. (eds.). *The collected papers of Otto Fenichel.* New York: Norton, 1954.

Freud, A. Problems of technique in adult analysis. *Bulletin of the Philadelphia Association for Psychoanalysis,* 1954, *4:* 44-70.

Freud, S. On narcissism, an introduction. In *Collected papers,* Vol. 14, London: Hogarth Press, 1914.

Freud, S. On psychotherapy. In *Collected papers.* Vol. I. London: Hogarth Press, 1924a.

Freud, S. Sexuality in the etiology of the neuroses. In *Collected papers.* Vol. I. London: Hogarth Press, 1924b.

Goldberg, A. Psychotherapy of narcissistic injuries. *Archives of General Psychiatry,* 1973, *28:* 722-726.

Goldfarb, A. I. The orientation of staff in a home for the aged. *Mental Hygiene,* 1953a, *8:* 343-347.

Goldfarb, A. I. Recommendations for psychiatric care in a home for the aged. *Jour nal of Gerontology,* 1953b, *8:* 343-347.

Goldfarb, A. I. Psychiatric problems of old age. *New York State Journal of Medicine, 1955a, 55:* 494-500.

Goldfarb, A. I. Psychotherapy of aged persons. IV. One aspect of the therapeutic situation with aged patients. *Psychoanalytic Review,* 1955b, *42:* 180-187.

Goldfarb, A. I. Psychotherapy with aged persons; patterns of adjustment in a home for the aged. *Mental Hygiene,* 1955c, *39:* 608-621.

Goldfarb, A. I. The rationale for psychotherapy with older persons. *American Journal of Medical Science,* 1956, *232:* 181-185.

Greenson, R. *The technique and pratice of psychoanalysis.* New York: International Universities Press, 1967.

Greenson, R. Beyond transference and interpretation. *International Journal of Psycho- analysis, 1972, 53, 213-217.*

Grotjahn, M. Psychoanalytic investigation of a seventy-one year old man with senile dementia. *Psychoanalytic Quarterly,* 1940, *9,* 80-97.

Grotjahn, M. Some analytic observations about the process of growing old. In Roheim, G. (ed.) *Psychoanalysis and social sciences.* Vol. 3. New York: Interna- tional Universities Press, 1951.

Grotjahn, M. Analytic psychotherapy with the elderly. *Psychoanaltyic Review,* 1955, *42:* 419-427.

Haley, J. *Problem-solving therapy.* San Francisco: Jossey-Boss, 1976.

Herr, J. and Weakland, J. *Counseling elders and their families.* New York: Springer, 1979.

Hollender, M. H. Individualizing the aged. *Social Casework,* 1952, 33: 337-342.

Jelliffee, S. E. The old age factor in psycho-analytic therapy. *Medical Journal Record,* 1925, 121: 7-12.

Jones, E. *The life and work of Sigmund Freud.* Vol. II. New York: Basic Books, 1957.

Kahana, R. Strategies of dynamic psychotherapy with the wide range of older in- dividuals. *Journal of Geriatric Psychiatry,* 1979, *12:* 71-100.

Kardiner, A. *The traumatic neuroses of war.* New York: Hoeber, 1941.

Karpf, R. J. Psychotherapy of depression with the elderly. *Psychotherapy: Theory, Research, Practice,* 1977, *14:* 349-353.

Karpf, R. J. Altering values via psychological reactance and reversal effects. *Journal of Social Psychology,* 1978, *106:* 131-132.

Karpf, R. J. Modalities of psychotherapy with the elderly. *Journal of the American Geriatrics Society,* 1980a, *28:* 367-371.

Karpf, R. J. Nonverbal components of the interpretive process in psychoanalytic psychotherapy. *American Journal of Psychotherapy,* 1980b, *34:* 477-486.

Khan, M. The concept of cumulative trauma. *Psychoanalytic Study of the Child,* 1963, *18:* 286-306.

Kohut, H. *The analysis of the self.* New York: International Universities Press, 1971.

Kris, E. Preconscious mental processes. *Psychoanalytic Quarterly,* 1950, *19:* 540-560.

Langs, R. *The therapeutic interaction.* Volume II. New York: Jason Aronson, 1976a.

Langs, R. *The bipersonal field.* New York: Jason Aronson, 1976b.

Lawton, G. Psychotherapy with older persons. *Psychoanalysis,* 1952, *1:* 27-41.

Lazarus, L. and Weinberg, J. Treatment in the ambulatory care setting. In Busse, E. and Blazer, D. (eds.) *Handbook of geriatric psychiatry.* New York: Van Nostrand Reinhold, 1980.

Lindeman, E. Symptomotology and management of acute grief. *American Journal of Psychiatry,* 1944, *101:* 101-112.

Low, A. *Mental health through will training.* Boston: Christopher, 1950.

Mahoney, M. J. *Cognition and behavior modification.* Cambridge, Mass.: Ballinger, 1974.

Malan, D. *A study of brief psychotherapy.* London: Tavistock Publications, 1963.

Malan, D. *The frontier of brief psychotherapy: An example of the convergence of research and clinical practice.* New York: Plenum Medical Book Company, 1976.

Marks, I. Behavioral psychotherapy of adult neuroses. In Garfield, S. and Bergin, A. (eds.) *Handbook of psychotherapy and behavior change: An empirical analysis.* New York: John Wiley, 1978.

Martin, L. J. *A handbook for old age counselors.* San Francisco: Geertz Printing Co., 1944.

Martin, L. J. and deGrunchy, C. *Salvaging old age.* New York: Macmillan, 1930.

Martin, L. J. and deGrunchy, C. *Sweeping the cobwebs.* New York: Macmillan, 1933.

Meerloo, J. Contribution of psychoanalysis to the problem of the aged. In Heiman, M. (ed.). *Psychoanalysis and social work.* New York: International Universities Press, 1953.

Meerloo, J. Psychotherapy with elderly people. *Geriatrics,* 1955a, *10:* 583-587.

Meerloo, J. Transference and resistance in geriatric psychotherapy. *Psychonanalytic Review,* 1955b, *42:* 72-82.

Parloff, M. Waskow, I., and Wolfe, B. Research on therapist variables in relation to process and outcome. In Garfield, S. and Bergin, A. (eds.) *Handbook of psychotherapy and behavior change.* New York: John Wiley, 1978.

Pincus, I. Reminiscence in aging and its implications for social work practice. In Steury, S. and Blank, M. (eds.) *Readings in psychotherapy with older people.* Rockville, Maryland: National Institute of Mental Health, 1977.

Pfeiffer, E. Psychotherapy with elderly patients. *Postgraduate Medicine,* 1971, *50:* 254-258.

Pfeiffer, E. and Busse, E. Mental disorders in later life—Affective disorders, paranoid, neurotic and situational reactions. In Busse, E. and Pfeiffer, E. (eds.). *Mental illness in later life.* Washington, D.C.: American Psychiatric Association, 1973.

Rechtschaffen, A. Psychotherapy with geriatric patients: a review of the literature. *Journal of Gerontology,* 1959, *14:* 73-89.

Ronch, J. and Maizler, J. Individual psychotherapy with the institutionalized aged. *American Journal of Orthopsychiatry,* 1977, *42:* 275-283.

Sandler, J. Countertransference and role-responsiveness. *International Review of Psychoanalysis,* 1976, *3:* 43-47.

Shapiro, A. K. and Morris, L. A. Placebo effects in medical and psychological therapies. In Garfield, S. and Bergin, A. (eds.). *Handbook of psychotherapy and behavior change: An empirical analysis.* New York: John Wiley, 1978.

Small, L. *The briefer psychotherapies*. New York: Brunner/Mazel, 1979.

Sparacino, J. Individual psychotherapy with the aged: A selective review. *International Journal of Aging and Human Development*, 1979, *9:* 197-220.

Verwoerdt, A. Training in geropsychiatry. In Busse, E. and Pfeiffer, E. (eds.). *Behavior and adaptation in late life*. Boston: Little, Brown, 1969.

Verwoerdt, A. *Clinical geropsychiatry*. Baltimore: Williams and Wilkins, 1976.

Weinberg, J. Psychiatric techniques in the treatment of older people. In Donahue, W. and Tibbitts, C. (eds.). *Growing in the older years*. Ann Arbor: University of Michigan Press, 1951.

Weinberg, J. Psychopathology. In Howells, J. (ed.). *Modern perspectives in the psychiatry of old age*. New York: Brunner/Mazel, 1975a.

Weinberg, J. Geriatric psychiatry. In Freedman, A., Kaplan, H., and Sadock, B. (eds.). *Comprehensive textbok of psychiatry*. Baltimore: Williams and Wilkins, 1975b.

Winnicott, D. *The maturational processes and the facilitating environment*. New York: International Universities Press, 1965.

Wolberg. L. R. (ed.). *Short-term psychotherapy*. New York: Grune and Stratton, 1965.

Wolff, K. *Geriatric psychiatry*. Springfield, Illinois: Thomas, 1963.

Wolff, K. *The emotional rehabilitation of the geriatric patient*. Springfield, Illinois: Thomas, 1970.

Zung, W. Affective disorders. In Busse, E. and Blazer, D. (eds.). *Handbok of geriatric psychiatry*. New York: Van Nostrand Reinhold, 1980.

3

Geriatric Group Psychotherapy

Arthur MacNeill Horton, Jr.
Maurice E. Linden

> It is the unusual event in medicine to find a single therapeutic
> agent that recommends itself as appropriately, offers supplies for
> as many needs, and manages the total person as felicitously as does
> group psychotherapy in the relief of the emotional disorders of later
> years. (Linden 1956, p. 129)

The purpose of this chapter will be to introduce the reader to group
psychotherapy with the aged. In order to provide the proper perspective, a
number of topics will need to be attended to. These will include the following areas. First, some consideration will be given to the special meaning of
the concept "group" in psychotherapy. Second, the historical background
of group psychotherapy with the aged will be surveyed. Third, a summary
of relevant research findings regarding outcome and process studies and
group psychotherapy with the elderly will be given. Fourth, attention will
be given to the practical clinical aspects of geriatric group management.
Major foci of interest will be stages of group development, leadership style
and group composition. These will be discussed with special reference to
aged individuals. Fifth, some case examples of group psychotherapy with
the elderly will be presented. Finally, some tentative conclusions with
regard to geriatric group psychotherapy will be offered.

This chapter was written by Arthur MacNeill Horton Jr. and Maurice E. Linden in their
private capacities. No official support or endorsement by the Veterans Administration is intended or should be inferred.

THE CONCEPT OF GROUP IN PSYCHOTHERAPY

It is noteworthy that Freud in his book, *Group Psychology and Analysis of the Ego,* averred that the number of patients was of no psychological significance and thus, there is no need to develop new concepts to explain the phenomena which occurs in group psychotherapy. Essentially, Freud's position implies that the group is merely a collection of individuals undergoing a common experience, and that the group may be perceived in terms of individual psychodynamics. In other words, group psychotherapy is seen as individual psychotherapy in a group setting.

A counter-view might be elucidated. Basically, it has been suggested that knowledge of individual psychodynamics is inadequate to explain the actual processes and behaviors which occur within the context of group psychotherapy. Put another way, people interacting with each other in a therapy group create a particular atmosphere and group culture which is only comprehensible by *both* understanding the psychology of the individuals involved and the sort of interpersonal environment their interactions have created. To a large degree, this second position owes something to the Gestalt Psychology postulate that the whole is more than the sum of its parts.

In terms of an overall statement regarding these two rather divergent viewpoints, the following is offered. Similarly, to his statement on the inappropriateness of the aged for psychotherapy, it may be asserted that Freud was mistaken on this point. By way of explanation, it might be recalled that the great analyst had done rather little group work. Perhaps, had Freud been involved in more group psychotherapy experiences, his keen clinical senses would have forced a revision of his first tentative impressions.

Rather clearly, many of the more recent group theorists make a distinction between a group and other classes of individuals. Krech and Crutchfield (1948) for instance, noted that a collection of Republicans or farmers is not a "group" per se. More realistically, they are "classes" of people. Indeed, the term "group" might more correctly be reserved for situations where two or more individuals have an interpersonal psychological relationship to each other. The fact that common language usage serves to obscure this psychological distinction should be fairly straightforward.

HISTORICAL BACKGROUND OF PSYCHOTHERAPY WITH THE AGED

In order to provide a historical perspective to better conceptualize group psychotherapy with the aged, the following remarks are offered.

Four major periods of group psychotherapy might be distinguished. These are early times to 1900; 1900 to 1930; 1930 to World War II; and from World War II to the present. Each will be briefly outlined.

Early times to 1900

Perhaps the earliest precursors of group psychotherapy were the primitive tribal rituals of cavemen. The war dances, and the council of elders are but two examples that spring to mind. In classical Greece, the Greek chorus, the forerunner of modern drama, provides an instance where group focuses were utilized. Moving forward to still more contemporary times, it is interesting to note that two rather controversial individuals were identified with the beginnings of group psychotherapy. For instance, Anton Mesmer, the hypnotist, held group sessions for his patients. Similarly, the infamous Marquis de Sade at the Asylum of Charenton conducted theatricals using mental patients as actors. It was believed that the plays had therapeutic benefit for the patients.

1900 to 1930

In the second period, the therapeutic values of group psychotherapy became more clearly realized by established mental health care professionals. The contributions of two individuals were of paramount importance. Largely, as a result of the efforts of J. H. Pratt and J. L. Moreno, group psychotherapy became a recognized therapeutic approach.

J. H. Pratt is generally considered to have been the first person to purposefully use group methods for therapeutic purposes (Gazda 1975). Pratt was a physician working in the Boston area. A few years after the turn of the century, Pratt decided to hold group meetings with tuberculosis patients for the purpose of saving time as he was instructing them in health practices. After a while, he found that those patients who were treated in groups did better than those seen individually. Thus, he began to appreciate the therapeutic value of a group, or as he referred to it, "class," approach (Pratt 1907).

J. L. Moreno is generally considered to be the father of group psychotherapy. Interestingly, he first began to use group psychotherapy while working with prostitutes in Vienna, Austria (Moreno 1966). In 1925, Moreno emigrated to the United States and in 1931 and 1932, introduced the terms *group therapy* and *group psychotherapy,* respectively (Gazda) 1975). By his many writings (Moreno 1934; Moreno and Toeman 1942; Moreno 1966), as well as organizational and editorial efforts, Moreno provided enterprising and creative leadership to the group psychotherapy movement (Gazda 1975).

1930 to World War II

In a similar manner but in a markedly different way from the previous period, the period from 1930 to World War II is symbolized by the contributions of two individuals. Two men, Paul Schilder and Samuel R. Slavson, integrated psychoanalytic procedures and group psychotherapy. This was no small task but clearly made group psychotherapy part of the mainstream of American mental health practice.

Paul Schilder was a psychoanalyst, who worked at Belleview Hospital in New York City. His reputation among his analytic colleagues was of the highest order. When Schilder began to use group methods and to write about them for leading professional journals (Schilder 1936), the use of groups for therapy became respectable and an accepted component of psychoanalytic thinking.

Samuel R. Slavson is best known for his development of "activity 'group therapy" (Gazda 1975). He was a prolific writer (Slavson 1943) and the editor of the *International Journal of Group Psychotherapy*. Slavson's leadership, to a large degree, served to further the wide-spread adoption of group techniques by mental health workers in America.

In sum, it might be said, psychoanalysis' incorporation of group methods may be primarily responsible for the great popularity of group psychotherapy.

World War II to Present

Since World War II, there has been a geometric increase in the growth of interest in and contributions to the field of group psychotherapy. Perhaps the major influence of the war was the creation of a situation where the needs of military psychiatry and psychology far outstripped the available mental health resources for providing the then traditional individual psychotherapy. Group psychotherapy was seen as allowing more patients to receive services. Thus, the human service needs secondary to war gave the group psychotherapy movement an impetus for growth. Among others, the work of W. R. Bion at the Northfields Military Hospital and later the Tavistock Clinic was of cardinal importance (Rosenbaum 1975).

Another major trend in the post-World War II period has been the inculcation of scientific findings from the fields of social psychology, sociology and anthropology. This literature has been termed "group dynamics" and deals with the scientific study of those interactive influences which arise in small group situations. Among others, the work of Lewin, Lippitt, Asch, and Sherif have been influential (Dinkmeyer and Muro 1971). The T-group approach of the National Training Laboratories (NTL) may be seen as an extension of the use of group dynamics for therapeutic purposes.

At this point, it might be freely admitted that an extensive review of the growth of group psychotherapy since World War II is beyond the scope of this chapter. Rather, in keeping with the overall intent of the chapter, further remarks will be devoted to specific developments relative to group psychotherapy with the elderly.

Quite remarkably, despite the long recognized value of participation by the elderly in group activities, there has been scant attention in the professional literature. Review chapters by Linden (1956) and Levy, Derogatis, Gallagher, and Gatz (1980) were able to identify very few studies. This is in sharp contrast to the great number of group participation and socialization programs sponsored by both governmental agencies and the voluntary sector. Given present day trends toward an increasing awareness of the needs of the elderly (Karpf 1978; Poon 1980), we could reasonably expect that group psychotherapy with the aging will be an area of increasing concern for mental health professionals.

PRACTICAL CLINICAL ASPECTS

In a very real sense, group therapy with the elderly is different than group therapy with other populations. Ralph Goldman, M.D. once remarked "the gerontologist is like a defeated general; he can't win against the effects of aging, so the best he can do is stage an orderly retreat." Thus, the very real age-related changes in mobility, sensory and cognitive abilities which characterize the elderly, provide a unique context for group therapy. The cognitive, affective, and behavioral problems of the elderly are particularly appropriate for group therapy as often the only aid that can be given is that of social and emotional support. For instance, to mention only two problems associated with the aging, dementia and depression, group therapy can play a role in ameliorating these cognitive and affective disorders. Often cases of mild dementia may be due to confusion. A reality orientation group (see Lewis, this volume) could be helpful in reorienting aged individuals. Similarly, the emotional support of group therapy can help the elderly cope with reactive depression secondary to a loss of somatic integrity. The point to remember is that while these problems may not be defeated still a certain quality of life can be maintained for the elderly individual through group therapy.

In the space alloted this chapter, it would not be possible to deal with all of the many clinical aspects relative to group psychotherapy for the elderly. Therefore, three overarching considerations will be selectively treated. These will be: stages of group development, leadership style, and group compositions. Hill(1971) has suggested that these three considerations determine what goes on in every therapy group.

Stages of Group Development

Rather surprisingly, there is a degree of consensus regarding the stages of group development. Very straightforwardly, four main stages can be identified. The following quote by Yalom very elegantly describes them:

> Broadly, groups go through an initial stage of orientation,

characterized by a search for structure and goals, a great dependency on the leader, and a concern about the group boundaries. Next, they encounter a stage of conflict, as the group deals with issues of interpersonal dominance. Following this, the group becomes increasingly concerned with intermember harmony and affection, while intermember differences are often submerged in the service of group cohesiveness. Much later, the fully developed work group emerges, which is characterized by high cohesiveness, considerable inter-and intrapersonal investigation, and full committedness to the primary task.

Interestingly, the four stages have been less eloquently described as "forming, storming, norming and conforming" or "flight, fight, insight, and love." It should be remembered that groups can move from one stage to another rather quickly and while there is a general progression towards forming a viable work group, there is no guarantee that all groups reach or pass through all stages. If anything, elderly groups might have a tendency to handle issues of interpersonal dominance in very well-socialized ways.

Leadership Style

In order to know what one needs to do, it is necessary to know where one wishes to go. One model for conceptualizing group processes is the Hill Interaction Matrix (Hill 1965; Hill 1971). This paradigm crosses the work style dimensions (responsive, conventional, assertive, speculative, and confrontive) and content styles (personal and relationship). Relative to therapy groups of elderly individuals, this schema, on its face, would appear to apply fairly well.

How one facilitates a group in achieving these desirable ends is a very difficult question. At this point in time, group leadership remains more of an art than a science. Still, some generalizations, gleamed from the authors' clinical experience in group therapy with geriatric patients will be provided. Three classes of group leader skills will be covered. These are management skills, caring skills and meaning attribution skills.

Management skills refer to the physical and verbal control of the group environment, both physical and psychological. Examples of relevant skills are structuring a discussion, gate keeping (keeping a discussion on a therapeutic issue and redirecting extraneous conversation) and setting limits on permissable behavior. In elderly groups, where one or two members may have a degree of organic brain impairment, the need for someone to do gate keeping would seem fairly straightforward. Similarly, the need to structure sessions according to the physical ability of members to pay attention is clear.

Caring skills refer to the affective dimension of group leadership. Indeed, if one wanted to fit the whole concept of group leadership skills into a convenient box, then one would say that management skills subserve the behavioral dimension and meaning attribution skills subserve the cognitive dimension so that when caring skills are added, one has a neat trinity of behavioral, affective, and cognitive components.

Discussion of three of these skills will provide a flavor of this dimension. "Tone setting" involves promoting a positive emotional climate with norms of cooperation, trust, and non-perfectionism. This is done by verbally and non-verbally positive reinforcement of action, words, or attitudes which support a helpful affective environment for the group (Thorensen and Potter 1975). Clearly, some limit-setting may be necessary in order that most interactions in geriatric group psychotherapy be positive. Interestingly, in the clinical experience of one of the authors, a ratio of at least three to one positive to negative affective comments is essential for a helpful emotional atmosphere in groups of elderly patients.

The other caring skills are sponsoring and tension relieving. Sponsoring involves encouraging a group member to interact or protecting a member from unproductive verbal assault. This skill is most valuable during the initial stages of group development when the potential for negatively charged interactions is greatest. Tension relieving refers to situations where the group is in a state of high anxiety or conflict and there is a need to reduce the level of tension so that productive work may proceed. Joking or calming are ways of allaying the anxiety of members and may redirect the group's energies into positive channels.

Meaning attribution skills refer to providing insight into their actions and relationships to the group. This is generally considered to be cognitively based. Four specific skills will be briefly discussed. The most elementary meaning attribution skill is, of course, giving information. For example, in geriatric groups, scientific information about age related changes could be helpful in correcting misconceptions. The myth about the inability of the aged to have sexual relations comes to mind as an instance where a specific bit of information could prove therapeutic. As most people are aware, interpretation or the proposing of tentative hypotheses for the probable causes of members' behavior is a traditional therapeutic technique and needs little explanation. Linking, however, is a less well known skill. When linking, one attempts to tie the similarities and differences of group members' interchanges together. For example, if one elderly man speaks about taking walks to combat boredom in a nursing home and another elderly woman talks about making handicrafts to pass the time, then the stage is set for the group therapist to identify a common problem which the group may wish to focus on and to illustrate various options for coping.

The last meaning attribution skill to be discussed is modeling. Essentially, this is the demonstration of appropriate behavior by role playing. The actual enactment of behavior has a unique therapeutic affect and a long tradition in group therapy (Moreno 1966). With elderly group members, it may have particularly powerful effects as there may be a slight tendency for many members to talk rather than do.

Group Composition

In terms of indications and contraindications for geriatric group psychotherapy, Linden (1956 pp. 141-142) suggested the following guidelines:

Positive Criteria

1. expressed desire to join the group
2. appearance of relative alertness
3. a fair degree of good personal hygiene
4. ability to understand English (or some language common to all of the group members)
5. ability to walk or be wheeled to meeting room
6. at least a minimal range of affects
7. evidence of some degree of adult adjustment prior to entrance into senile state
8. capacity for evoking interest and affection from nursing and attendant personnel
9. sardonic hostility

Negative Criteria

1. dementia (severe, unreversable)
2. advanced physical debility
3. systematized and chronic paranoid thought life
4. manic behavior
5. intense chronic hostility with assaultiveness
6. unremitting bowel and bladder incontinence
7. advanced deafness
8. monothematic hypochondriasis
9. undirected restlessness with inability to sit still
10. unwillingness to participate
11. inability to understand English (or some language common to all of the group members)

The above criteria, however, should be applied in an intuitive clinical manner and not used as inflexible rules.

While there is a long standing issue on whether psychotherapy groups should be "homogeneous or heterogeneous" the only generally accepted conclusion is that homogeneous groups, *in general,* are easier to work with. A better question might be posed as "homogeneous for what vs heterogeneous for what." While different authorities give diverse opinions, clinical wisdom suggests that very disturbed individuals, such as psychotic or severely demented patients, who may get little out of the group interaction and who will, on the other hand, hinder the development of a therapeutic atmosphere in the group, might be excluded. The crucial point seems to be that each group member should be able to profit from the group experience while not preventing others from profiting from the group experience.

A method for ascertaining this information has been referred to as the "group reaction" or "trial group" approach. Essentially, a pilot group experience is conducted and then a decision is made on the basis of actual group behavior (Yalom 1975). This method has a number of advantages but may prove difficult to implement in some clinical settings. For example, it would be difficult to solicit patients in a nursing home if the therapist was unable to assure them a definite group experience.

Group therapists should be cognizant of the group balance. That is, the individuals that are included shouldn't all be the sort who would form a group norm which will go counter to the direction the therapist wishes to go. For example, if all of the elderly individuals in a group are apathetic and withdrawn, it is difficult to see how a group norm of activity and social interaction could easily develop. It would be better to compose a group when two-thirds of the group of elderly individuals are relatively active and social and one third are apathetic and withdrawn. One would expect that a greater number of active individuals are relatively active and social and one third are apathetic and withdrawn. One would expect that a greater number of active individuals will force a group norm of activity and social interaction and they will exert group pressure on the less active individuals to change their behavior. The function of the therapist will be to see that the group pressure is exerted in a therapeutic manner. In composing a therapy group, one wishes to "stack the deck" in the direction one wishes to go.

The final point refers to group size. It has been suggested that the maximum number of participants in a therapy group is sixteen (Dinkmeyer and Muro, 1971). That is an absolute maximum, however, and the average group is probably eight to ten members. This, of course, should vary with the cognitive skills of the group members. It is possible to imagine circumstances which would dictate a geriatric psychotherapy group of three to five members. The decision the clinician has to make is when the group works, and generally the smaller the size, the more control over group process the therapist has. If some geriatric group members have a mild degree of dementia and thus may have difficulty concentrating upon the group discourse, it may be helpful to have a small group so the therapist can ensure that each group member is fully involved.

Establishing and Maintaining the Group

After the environmental aspects such as the physical setting and furniture have been decided, a question arises how to get the group "going." (Of course, with the aging, often the need for wheel chair access and sound proofing are sailent). While any simplistic answer will prove futile in a significant number of cases, one concrete suggestion might be offered. Often group exercises may serve to "break the ice" in an initial group meeting. Activities as simple and harmless as asking everyone to, in turn, repeat each group member's name can serve to reduce emotional discomfort and promote a positive helpful but nonperfectionistic climate. A series of exercises (Dinkmeyer and Muro 1971) were developed for children but can be adpated to the elderly with some fairly straightforward modifications.

The developing understanding of self and others (DUSO) series, which is based upon Adlerian Psychology, has a number of group exercises that are useful for promoting group cohesion. One of the authors has used these exercises with groups of elderly patients with some success. One of the exercises, designed for the first group meeting, involves having a group member give his or her name, then the next group member gives the name of the person who went before him or her and the next group member must give the names of both individuals as well as his or her name and so on with each group member taking a turn. This serves as an effective introduction and insures that all group members will know each other's names. Linden (1956) has described aging as "childhood in reverse" and it would seem that a number of modifications of group procedures, such as explicit limits, small group size, and shortened group meeting time may be appropriate for some elderly individuals. As there is a wealth of literature on group therapy for children, which contrasts with a paucity of literature on group therapy for the elderly, the former might be consulted for further suggestions. It is, of course, recognized that the group therapist must be sensitive to the dignity of his or her aged patients and not use materials that might prove insulting to an elderly person.

RESEARCH

Unfortunately, group psychotherapy with the elderly appears to be an area which has received scant attention from psychotherapy researchers. In a recent definitive chapter on group research (Bednar and Kaul 1978) *not one* of either of the process or outcome studies reviewed *used elderly individuals* as subjects. Thus, it would seem one's clinical experience may not be necessarily the best but rather the only guide available.

The major problem in psychotherapy research is the lack of clinically sensitive but scientifically respectable outcome measures (Yalom 1975).

This puzzle is continuing and is multiplied in group therapy by the complexity of the phenomena under study (Bednar and Kaul 1978).

Regarding the overall worth of group therapy, Bednar and Kaul (1978) conclude that:

> It is safe to conclude that selected group treatments are useful, even though our knowledge about the limits of the usefulness are embarrassingly limited. (p. 810)

In short, group therapy will continue to be on shaky scientific ground until the fundamental phenomena have been identified and systematically studied. Unfortunately, these are puzzles that will require much additional work in the future.

CONCLUSIONS

It is suggested here that geriatric group psychotherapy be considered a *valuable method of treatment for the aged.* Its potential contribution to the social and psychological welfare of the increasing aged population in the United States must be considered quite great. At a time when loneliness, confusion, and disorientation may be increasing threats to emotional health, positive social support from the group situation can be a godsend to elderly individuals. Its potential contribution to the social and psychological welfare of the increasing aged population must be considered quite great. As observed by Linden (1956):

> Group psychotherapy with the aged is being employed increasingly in many institutions throughout the country. Considered in terms of relief of suffering alone, it is well worth the effort it entails. But its promise is greater than that. It affords an area of study which may confirm or amend present psychiatric concepts, thus indirectly benefiting younger age groups. It may help to demonstrate that there is a potential for mental development continuously through life even into the later years. And it may contribute to that very necessary long-term culture-wide endeavor directed toward returning to the elders a measure of veneration to the end that even the sunset of life may contain an invigorating social reward. It is quite likely that when human existance becomes meaningful at its every turning, then many of the now extant forms of so-called senility will be relics of the past (p. 151).

CASE STUDIES

These case studies were selected to provide a clinical appreciation of the subtle personality changes engendered by group psychotherapy with the elderly. An important point in all of these case studies is that the social and emotional support provided by group psychotherapy with their age peers gave them an increased appreciation of the positive aspects of interpersonal relationships.

Case I: Problems of Daily Living

This elderly woman was experiencing multiple difficulties in the activities of daily living. Group therapy was able to reawaken her interest in life after two years of treatment. By helping others to gain insight, she apparently benefited herself.

Case I, E. M. This married woman was sixty-five at the time of admission to the state hospital. All her life she had been healthy and happy. Following several years of employment as an elite domestic, at the age of forty-four she married a widower with two children. She was described as obstinate, quick-tempered, but able to give and take jokes. She was thorough and neat. Nothing of her childhood was known to informants. Her admission to the hospital was occasioned by her being nervous, worried about money, agitated, depressed, and upset about her memory, her health, her husband, and her finances." She asked of the admitting physician, "Did you ever feel like you had sinned?" For two years of hospitalization, she remained restless, anxious, retarded, depressed, and even too frightened to accept privileges. She began attending group psychotherapy on the advice of her physician. There her memory showed spotty impairment, but, except for her melancholic mood, most of her mental faculties were fairly intact. Her transference in therapy was classified as predominantly negative, hostile-depressed. Her improvement in group psychotherapy was steady and very slow. Within a year, she was able to accept increasing freedoms. Later, she became cautiously cheerful. In early 1952, she began making home visits. She was a passive participant in group psychotherapy at the beginning, but months later, she started talking about her childhood and living experiences. As her diffidence fell away, she proceeded to demonstrate a fairly remarkable understanding of human nature and helped others gain insights as she prospered. Her transference turned warm and friendly as time passed. Interestingly, at this point, her psychological tests and evaluations showed normal mood, memory, and capabilities. She left the hospital after two years. Interim reports reveal that she is leading a normal community life and has been working as a domestic in order to help with the family finances. Her husband described her very recently as "even better than when she left the hospital."

Case II: Delusions

The aged woman demonstrated rather bizzare delusions. Group therapy provided an arena where she could work through her repressed sexual feelings and gain insight into her frustration. After three years of group therapy, she was able to rid herself of her delusions and assume a more adjusted social role.

Case II, M. L. When admitted at age seventy, this short, very stout woman was said to have shown signs of mental illness for many years. She complained that a neighbor placed a copperhead snake in her bed and that other snakes inhabited the cellar. She heard voices giving her commands she had to follow. Restless and disturbed at night, she remained in bed all day. There was no informant acquainted with her early history. She had been living as something of a recluse for several years. On examination, she showed evidence of preservation of intellect and most psychological modalities except in the areas of mental illness. During about seven years of hospitalization, the patient was a noisy and militant ward tyrant. Embittered, seclusive, paranoid, and argumentative, she was disliked by patients and personnel. One day, she wrote to her ward physician.

> Perhaps it would interest you to know that I am a Freemail with Mail eyes. You should see the X-ray pictures taken of me. One doctor thinks I have two hearts. If one lets go the other would take over. I only feel one beating. But I have just about two of everything else inside. Two sets of intestines and two stomachs, one inactive and glad of it for it is hard to supply one stomach let alone two. I am such a medical freak.

In group psychotherapy this patient's keen intellect became a pivotal reference point. Her comprehensions of others' needs were precise, accurate, and searching. She recounted her own dreams, hallucinations, and delusions and gave valuable associations which led to insight formation and a good deal of working through. A dramatic turning point took place in therapy one day when she suddenly confessed to the group that she was a frustrated spinster whose sexual longings were always disappointed and that "even today, and you may not believe it because I'm seventy-nine, I have hopes that the right man will come along and marry me." Unable to leave the hospital permanently because of physical limitations due to obesity, M. is now a charming, affable, cheerful, and cooperative woman whose letters are coherent and without a shred of dereistic fantasy. She has been in group psychotherapy continuously for three years. No manifestations of psychosis are present. A volunteer visitor has taken a liking to the patient and has had M. to her home for many visits up to five days in length. The patient is now eighty years old.

Case III: Memory Loss

The elderly widow presented a fairly pronounced impairment of memory. Social and emotional support from the group therapy sessions provided a reason for her to become more alert and oriented. After one year, the woman had improved so much that return to the community was contemplated.

Case III, E.L.L. This eighty-six year old widow was admitted with the following commitment statements, "This patient shows loss of memory for recent events and confusion. She is uncertain whether or not she owns property, is unable to tell the street address where she lives and how long she has lived there." She believed that her relatives were being substituted by strangers. Quarrelsome, periodically agitated, and careless and untidy in personal hygiene, the patient developed the notion that everyone was against her. Psychological tests showed the impairments common to "senility." Clinically, the patient was described as wizened and enfeebled. Following her entrance into the group psychotherapy (delayed because of hospital treatment for several physical ailments), Mrs. L. became very effective as a ward worker, gained weight, and became noticeably robust and cheerful. This was due in no small measure to her medical and surgical treatment. However, in group participation, she became progressively oriented, filled in many memory hiati, and frequently volunteered recitations, whereas earlier she had been very shy, perplexed, and withdrawn. At the present time, this patient's daughter is considering removing her eighty-eight year-old mother to her home. The patient is now nearly fully oriented and alert. Bowel and bladder incontinence, which were present the first nine months of hospital stay, have been absent completely after one year of treatment.

Case IV: Depressed State

The aged woman had been severely depressed for an extended period of time. Group therapy, combined with appropriate medication, enabled this woman to make a dramatic change in her affective adjustment after only a few months. In all probability, her relationship with the male therapist was a primary factor for the improvement shown.

Case IV, F. R. This elderly widow is a remarkable case. She spent nearly twelve miserable years in a bitter, hostile, passively depressed state after being admitted at age sixty-five. She was self-isolated, self-recriminatory, unconsolably vituperative and hotly sarcastic. Institutional life was for her an empty unpleasantness. She showed enthusiasm and ambition only for death. She was placed on a stimulating drug routine and after two months, when she was sufficiently alert and apparently hungry for social contacts, she was coerced into attending group therapy. There she showed a pseudo-rejecting transference and in a few months she became affable, jocular, teasing, and beneficently wily. She actually fell deeply in love with the male therapist, asked to kiss him, and twittered and blushed like a virginal adolescent whenever he came near. She gained weight, became much more agile, and proved to be a witty raconteur in group meetings. Her emotional interplay with the other participants in a web of positive transference efforts to gain the therapist's favor was an unsurpassed experience for all observers. Mrs. R. developed a tranquility and good humor she had not known for a sixth of her life. She would walk about the building singing and saying encouraging things to other patients. Many months later she died of a known heart ailment only after she had proved conclusively that group psychotherapy with the aged is a potent therapeutic agent. Her passing was an occasion for mourning among all the patients and personnel who had known her through the therapeutic period.

References

Burrett, C. Effectiveness of widow's groups in facilitating change. *Journal of Consulting and Clinical Psychology*, 1978, *46*, 20-31.

Bednar, R. L. & Kaul, T. J. Experiential group research: current perspectives. In S. Garfield & A. Bergin (eds.) *Handbook of psychotherapy and behavior change*, (2nd Ed.). New York: Wiley, 1978.

Dinkmeyer, D. C. & Muro, J. J. *Group counseling: theory and practice.* Itasca, Illinois: F. E. Peacock, 1971.

Gallagher, P. Comparative effectiveness of group psychotherapies for the reduction of depression in elderly outpatients. Paper presented at the meeting of the American Psychological Association, New York, August, 1979.

Gazda, G. M. (ed) *Basic approaches to group psychotherapy and group counseling*, (2nd Ed.). Charles C. Thomas: Springfield, Illinois, 1975.

Hill, W. F. *Hill interaction matrix.* Los Angeles: University of Southern California Youth Study Center, 1965.

Hill, W. F. The Hill interaction matrix. *Personnel and Guidance Journal*, 1971, *49*, 619-623.

Ingersoll, B. & Silverman, A. Comparative group psychotherapy for the aged *Gerontologist*, 1978, *18*, 201-206.

Karpf, R. J. Some observations on a trend towards geriatrics in clinical psychology. *Professional Psychology*, 1978, *9*, 672-676.

Keller, J. & Croake, J. Effects of a program in rational thinking on anxieties in older persons. *Journal of Counseling Psychology*, 1975, *22*, 54-57.

Krech, D. & Crutchfield, R. S. *Theory and Problems of Social Psychology.* New York: McGraw-Hill, 1948.

Levy, S. M., Derogatis, L. R., Gallagher, D., & Gatz, M. Intervention with older adults and the evaluation of outcome. In L. Poon (ed.) *Aging in the 1980's.* Washington, D.C.: American Psychological Association, 1980.

Linden, M. E. Group psychotherapy with institutionalized senile women. *International Journal of Group Psychotherapy*, 1953, *3*, 150.

Linden, M. E. Geriatrics. In S. R. Slavson (ed.) *The fields of group psychotherapy.* New York: International Universities Press, 1956.

Moreno, J. L. *Who shall survive.* Washington, D.C.: Nervous and Mental Diseases Publishing Co., 1934.

Moreno, J. L. & Toeman, Z. The group approach in psychodrama. *Sociometry*, 1942, *5*, 191-196.

Moreno. J. L., et al. (eds.) *The international handbook of group psychotherapy.* New York: Philosophical Library, 1966.

Poon, L. (ed.) *Aging in the 1980's.* Washington, D.C.: American Psychological Association, 1980.

Pratt, J. H. The class method of treating consumption in the homes of the poor. *Journal of the American Medical Association,* 1907, *49,* 755-757.

Rosenbaum, M. Group psychotherapy and psychodrama. In B. Wolman, *Handbook of clinical psychology.* pp. 1254-1274. New York: McGraw-Hill, 1965.

Schilder, P. The analysis of ideologies as a psychotherapeutic method, especially in group treatment. *American Journal of Psychiatry,* 1936, *93,* 601-618.

Thoresen, C. E. and Potter, B. Behavioral Group Counseling. In G. M. Gazda (ed). *Basic Approaches to Group Psychotherapy and Group Counseling.* Springfield, Illinois: Charles C. Thomas, 1975.

Yalon, I. *The theory and practice of group psychotherapy.* New York: Basic Books, 1975.

Part Two
Innovative Psychotherapeutic Approaches

4

Absence of Purposeful Behavior: Issues in Training the Profoundly Impaired Elderly

Robert W. Kennedy
Ann B. Kennedy

Despite all the recent attention to the older population, there remains at least one group of individuals unaffected by this upsurge of interest. For the purposes of this chapter, this group will be labelled after the most visible characteristic of its members, the apparent absence of purposeful behavior (APB). Since this is a descriptive rather than standardized diagnostic term, some deliberation must be given to a working definition of the traits and behavior included under this rubric.

The operational definition of absence of purposeful behavior here refers to functional level rather than to a demographic or diagnostic category. Where most classification schemes can be seen as vertical, with a number of disorders or problems described but allowing for a range of severity (depth) for each, the choice of a horizontal scheme is made only with a view to treatment considerations, which in this case correspond to severely depressed levels of functioning that cut across classes of causation.

Though APB encompasses, frequently, a great number of symptoms, disorders and behaviors, there is only one necessary trait, the nearly total lack of self-preserving or self-care behavior. These people, it is usually observed, simply don't do very much of anything. Although they are functionally quite impaired, and seem not to respond to most training or therapeutic interventions, it is our primary premise that this is a treatable problem that does not, for the most part, depend upon the etiology of the disorder, but rather upon staff awareness of motivational variables and use of appropriate treatment techniques.

Individuals exhibiting APB are likely to show deficits in all areas of functioning. Among the cognitive functions (e.g., orientation, memory, attention, calculation and language) spontaneous production may be nil, and even formalized mental status examination will elicit few, if any, appropriate responses. Regardless of diagnosis, such responses are indistinguishable from those found in cases of severe organic mental disorders. Behaviorally, these people do not care for themselves in any of the usual activities of daily living (ADL), and are invariably classified as requiring total nursing care. Repetitive, apparently unproductive actions, such as rocking, pacing (when ambulatory) or moaning are fairly common, as are incontinence and seemingly randomly directed aggression. Social behavior is almost non-existent. Affect is noticeable either in its absence or in a kind of hyperexcited state that mimics agitation or distress. Due to limitations in cognition and self-expression, no assessment of sensory impairment is possible, and symptoms of medical problems are quite difficult to identify.

The causes of APB are many, but the most common are probably senile or pre-senile dementia, cerebrovascular disturbance, organic mental disorder (most frequently due to alcohol intoxication), and possibly cerebral arteriosclerosis. It is the authors' opinion that there is invariably an iatrogenic, or institution-caused, component that interacts with one or more medical problems to produce the extreme levels of impairment seen in the APB syndrome. At the risk of oversimplifying, we postulate that there is an assumption by health care workers that the locus of the disorder is entirely within the individual, that it cannot be reversed, and therefore no significant positive change can be expected from such individuals. This produces, more or less directly, the unquestioning over-caring that contributes to the total dependence so often observed. The severity of the medical conditon, combined with complete dependence and the inability to communicate satisfactorily interact to create feelings of total alienation from the APB client—alienation so pronounced that workers are blinded to the fact that the client is a human being. This, in turn, leads to further dehumanizing treatment practices, and perpetuates the APB stereotype by completing the vicious cycle.

Readers who have worked in most chronic care institutions will recognize clients characterized by APB as the minority relegated to the back wards, the units where feeding, sleeping, bathing and behavior control occupy the entire day, where professional staff rarely make an appearance, and where staff morale is often the lowest in the institution. They will also recognize that these are the clients least likely to have benefited from reality orientation or remotivation programs, even when such apparently potent reinforcers as popular staff, profuse attention, family visits, or favorite foods are used. This is an especially devastating experience for workers who have been willing to persevere in helping those who are labelled, by the "common wisdom," as unhelpable. Even whittling one's expectations down to a minimal level seems not to help.

MAJOR POINTS IN TREATING APB

There are three issues to be addressed in any successful approach to working with clients who exhibit the APB syndrome. The first of these relates to staff attitudes, and must be considered of primary importance, since without positive expectations and a belief in a worthwhile, dignified existence for clients with severe impairment, no worker will expend the intensive effort required to produce behavior change. There is no better or more lasting way to engender appropriate attitudes than to demonstrate the success of a particular technique, and methods that can be employed by as few as one or two workers obviates the need for sweeping—and unlikely—institutional changes. It is true that health care settings are as prone to the absence of purposeful behavior as the patients we are discussing; for change to occur, goals have to be achievable, staff expectations must be positive but realistic, and methods need to be appropriate to the institution's resources for the task to be accomplished. Institutional behavior is only a function of the actions of its individual members, so we accept as axiomatic that real change comes only through the growth of individuals. And, if this seems to be a tedious process, it will pay to remember that at least it can be accomplished without the usual frustrating, time consuming and often unsuccessful bureaucratic wrangling.

A second problem is the choice of appropriate skills or tasks with which to work. Institutional staff may identify a number of self-care skills such as self-feeding, toileting and dressing which they believe to be of the highest priority. Close examination of staff wishes, however, may reveal that the skills are chosen because of potential benefit to staff, rather than the client. In the best of all possible worlds, only skills that the client both wants and needs would be taught, for this conforms to the ideal notion of what should take place in any treatment setting. Realistically, however, treatment staff often wish to teach clients to do things that either reduce staff work load or diminish behaviors (e.g., incontinence) that others find objectionable. Inasmuch as there is a close correspondence between staff desires and what the client must be able to do (and is willing to learn) to provide maximally independent self-care in the least restrictive environment, this presents no difficulty. When the client is likely to remain in the present institution, the problem becomes increasingly apparent. From the client's point of view, there may be no compelling reason to change, particularly since he or she may feel quite depressed about the loss of function and yet comfortable in a near-complete state of dependency. It is beyond the scope of this chapter to consider all the possible variations of these and other motivational factors, but it must be realized that there may be a gulf between staff and client expectations which needs to be breached if staff expertise and client perseverence are to be allies in the treatment/training process. Lack of meaningful communication, a major difficulty with APB clients, hinders this process. A tendency on the part of workers to assume that there really isn't much going on mentally is extremely dangerous, for it may lead to further dehumanization. Yet, even assuming that the client is capable of rational, responsible thought, one cannot directly ascertain the nature of his/her motivations. Forced to live with this most unhappy ambiguity, we must nevertheless remain sensitive to cues from our clients that not only indicate a response to treatment, but which also reveal their wishes regarding the direction such training may take.

The type of skills to be learned are, of course, dependent on the factors mentioned in the prior discussion. Within those confines, however, there are a vast range of activities, many of which are rarely if ever offered to the elderly. Since many characteristics of the APB client are similar to those of other severely handicapped individuals (e.g., the mentally retarded), we believe that the basic programs for the handicapped delineated by Williams, Brown and Certo (1976) are appropriate for the APB client as well. The skills listed below have been modified somewhat from the Williams et al., listing in order to increase their suitability for the elderly.

Sensori-Motor Integration

1. Responding to signals, warnings
2. Discriminating distances, locations, temperatures

Recreation and Leisure

1. Modified golf, bowling, independent walking
2. Card playing, board games
3. Use of radio, record player, television, camera

Self-Care for Increased Independence

1. Selecting foods at mealtime and snacks
2. Snack and meal preparation
3. Using appropriate eating utensils
4. Using small appliances (can and bottle openers, shaver)
5. Bathing and showering, shampooing
6. Applying deodorant
7. Shaving
8. Combing, brushing, blow-drying, setting hair
9. Choosing clothing, dressing
10. Using toilet independently and privately

11. Self-medication

Communication

1. Using the telephone
2. Using gestures when needed
3. Expressing opinions, wishes
4. Letter writing, card signing

Community

1. Using the public telephone
2. Using public transportation with assistance, if needed
3. Protective skills (responding to street lights, warning signs)
4. Money skills (buying goods, a ticket to a movie, etc.)

The third major issue concerns the general approach and specific methods to be used with APB clients. We believe that a most fruitful approach lies in a combination of attribution theory based approach to motivation and behavioral technology.

Attribution theorists (Weiner 1974; Weiner, Frieze, Kukla, Reed, Rest and Rosenblaum 1972) state that achievement is most frequently attributed to one or more of four factors: effort, ability, task difficulty and luck. The first two, effort and ability, are internal to the achiever; task difficulty and luck are external, lying outside the individual. Also, consider that ability and task difficulty are relatively stable, while luck and effort are not. The two by two grid formed by the four factors on these two dimensions provides a basis for explaining perceptions of causation and also the responses of both the achiever and external observers to behavior. Attributions (which can also be called self-statements about cause and effect relationships) may themselves act as determinants of future behavior by forming a belief system that predetermines one's responses in certain situations. As we will see, they may be the basis of a negative self-image that exacerbates the APB syndrome.

In general, the amount of reinforcement offered, other things being equal, will be highest as task difficulty and the individual's efforts increase. When a task is seen as achievable due to luck or to the achiever's inherent ability, reinforcement will probably diminish. Of course, the reverse will also be true, with little reinforcement being extended for less effort and/or task difficulty, while perceptions of limited ability and/or luck will result in a higher probability of reinforcement.

Translated into practical terms, this means that climbing Mt. Everest (high effort and task difficulty) is likely to bring much social reinforcement, while winning a million dollar lottery (luck) or fixing breakfast (no challenge for one of average ability) should bring no particular reward.

How does this apply to work with APB clients? Since we are referring primarily to the learning of basic ADL skills and recreational activities, quite common tasks that are accomplished by most people with little difficulty, luck does not really affect the outcome. For the most part, task difficulty can also be ruled out as a significant factor, since both the client and the worker "know," from past experience, that these are among the easiest tasks in normal living. This leaves ability and effort as the salient variables in the attributional schema.

When an APB client is given social reinforcement by health care workers for accomplishing some previously easy ADL task, instead of increasing the prospect that the task will be performed again, they may inadvertantly be decreasing the probability. The client, having just been through the experience, knows that it is no longer easy, and the increased effort required conveys the message that his or her abilities are now marginally adequate at best. The "reinforcement" by treatment staff may only communicate that they, too, are aware of these inadequacies. Phrased another way, what is being positively reinforced is the client's low self image, rather than his performance improvement. The paucity of direct communication makes reinforcement an even riskier proposition, for, with the exception of carefully measured performance changes, the worker has no direct way of knowing what effect this is having on the client.

When in doubt, it is probably better to supply no contingent reinforcement that can be construed as placing a value on the client as a person. Noncontingent (unconditional) approval of the client as a human being cannot be harmful, and is almost always a positive motivating force. Similarly, contingent approval of a particular behavior or group of behaviors is quite helpful in retraining of ADL and recreational skills. The difficulty for many workers is in discriminating reinforcers that are "helpful" in changing the desired behavior from those that imply (either directly or through distortions by the client) an evaluation of personal worth.

For example, in training dressing skills, a simple "O.K." or "right" conveys a specific message, such as "you put your left arm in the correct sleeve." (Of course, this assumes a precise timing of reinforcing feedback to the exact moment of response.) It is difficult to imagine any negative attributional self-statements that a client might construct from the trainer's remark. On the other hand, giving the client candy or exclaiming what a wonderful job he or she is doing may, while conceivably producing the desired learning, also reinforce negative attributional self-statements. The client may learn to accept this reinforcement without protest, but it may be at a high cost in terms of self-image, infantilization, and a new dependency—this time on the institutional reward system.

Both the outcome (skill or other learning) and process (teaching methods, reinforcement) are fraught with potential attributional pitfalls.

Only by considering in advance the precise skill to be taught and the methods to be used can most of these be avoided. Since our clientele is not very helpful in this process, it is better to be safe than sorry. If the skill has no immediate use or is trite, don't teach it; if a reinforcer or method can be construed as childish or demeaning, don't use it. Thorough knowledge of the individual's former lifestyle, as a key to closely held values, family relationships, and reactions to previous treatment attempts can supply important information. Finally, an empathetic approach—being willing to put oneself in the patient's shoes—will reveal many common treatment practices (particularly in the verbal mode) that are quite demeaning.

In the area of learning, the aging field is, to date, still quite constricted. Most of what has been researched deals with learning in normal aging or with individuals suffering only mild impairment; very little has been said about learning and the severely impaired elderly. In his review of the research literature, Botwinick (1978) concluded that the elderly perform less well than younger subjects on most learning tasks. Performance has been augmented, in most cases, by slowing the pace of learning, providing more meaningful tasks (certainly relevant to the preceding discussion of attribution theory), and reducing autonomic arousal associated with disruptive emotional states (p. 305). Performance tends to be lowered by interference from stimuli or events (internal or external) during or following learning, attempting to do more than one task, or simultaneous stimulation by more than one source (p. 296). There is some evidence that old habits interfere with the acquisition of new ones (p. 300). In broad perspective, it appears that we are reconfirming what has always been accepted as "common sense": people slow down as they age; the more events that occur simultaneously, the harder it is to attend to the task at hand; people do best what they like to do; anxiety interferes with learning. These generalized, replicated findings, while not specific to the APB syndrome, do apply to retraining programs. In fact, such principles apply more to this population than to most others, due to the severity of their disability. Unfortunately, most research has failed to come to grips with this problem, either by ignoring APB clients or by using treatment techniques that do not incorporate these factors.

In assessing the behavior therapy literature, Richards and Thorpe (1978) reported very few studies dealing with APB. There were some positive findings in the areas of self-care and personal hygiene, but most studies were limited in scope or sophistication (pp. 262-264). Many potential resources, such as the intensive treatment of incontinence by Azrin, Sneed and Foxx (1973) have not yet found wide application. Storandt et al., concluded that the behavioral techniques which have proven successful with younger populations have also worked with the elderly, where they have been tried. They note also that most problems dealt with have been chosen by staff, and reflect their wishes to remove some form of objectionable behavior, rather than the more positive method of retraining specific competencies.

A more utilitarian approach to dealing with retraining is found in the field of mental retardation, which has generated many skill training programs more suited to the optimistic outlook of competency-centered (versus problem-centered) treatment. Some of these can be easily adapted to the requirements of APB clients.

Perhaps the most publicized of these programs is that designed by Gold (1975) and his colleagues for institutionalized, profoundly retarded clients. This approach, referred to as "Try Another Way," is based on a philosophy of the dignity and the right to choose of the individual, and presupposes that treatment failure is due to a lack of "power" in training techniques rather than the inherent limitations of the client. He uses a series of steps to define a skill to be trained, the method to be used, and a task analysis to break the behavior into teachable units.

For the purposes of this chapter, we will deal primarily with a task analysis approach as a means of preparing the staff and client for learning a predesignated skill. The task analysis approach enables the worker to become intimately familiar with the skills to be taught, and in so doing, develops an empathetic feeling for the client as he or she learns the skill.

The first step in developing a task analysis is clearly defining the skill to be taught, or what is also called the terminal objective. This objective or goal answers the following questions. What will the client be able to do on completion of training? Where will the client perform the skill and under what conditions? How often will the client perform this skill?

Using an example of learning to put on a belt, the terminal objective might be stated as follows:

> Each day, after putting on his socks, underwear, shirt and pants, the client will take his belt from the closet and put it on, correctly buckling it.

This objective assumes, of course, that the client can already put on socks, underwear, shirt and pants. Thus, putting on the belt might be the final step in a general dressing program; or, perhaps the client's appearance is always unkempt and he simply never remembers his belt. The assumption that he or she can dress, except for the belt, is referred to as an entering skill. In other words, the entering skill is the behavior that the client can do acceptably well at the beginning of this training.

Another example of a terminal objective, this time for using a napkin, might be:

> At each meal, after every few bites of food, the client will lift his or her napkin from the lap, wipe his or her mouth so that no food or liquid

remains on the face, and replace the napkin.

In this case, the entering skill is independent eating.

Once the objective of training is clearly established, the next step is the actual analysis of the task or skill. In simple terms, the skill is merely broken into a temporal sequence of small enough steps that it can be taught to the client. Returning to the belt example, these steps might be as follows:

1. Hold the belt by the plain (non-buckled) end with the dominant hand.
2. Push it through the belt loop.
3. Pull the plain end through the loop to the next loop with the non-dominant hand.
4. Push the belt through the next loop with the dominant hand (analysis continues through the final, or buckling, steps)

Although this may seem to be a slow and cumbersome process, it is more reliable than teaching by the usual method of verbal direction, demonstration, and then relying on the client to fumble around until the task is completed or until he or she simply gives up. In fact, if after task analysis the client still omits or performs a step incorrectly, it may be necessary to break the original steps into still smaller increments. Step 1 (above) might, for example, require further refinement into five segments:

1. Extend fingers on dominant hand.
2. Move hand over the plain end of the belt.
3. Lower hand onto the belt.
4. Grasp the plain end of belt.
5. Lift the belt end to the position of the first loop.

Of course, with clients whose current functioning does not require fine gradations in the task analysis, several steps may be combined for more efficient training and to avoid boring the client.

A task can be further analyzed by delineating the same steps in terms of what both the worker and the client should do. To illustrate, consider the five fine steps just discussed:

What the Worker Does:

1. Gently move the dominant hand of the client and while holding it with one hand, flex the fingers down from the wrist so that they extend naturally.

2. Gently move the client's hand

What the Client Does

1. Extend fingers of the dominant hand.

2. Move the hand over to the

over to the plain end of the
belt and point to the place on
the belt where the client is to
put his hand.

plain end of belt.

3. Gently move the client's hand
   down to the belt, pointing to
   the belt.

3. Lower the hand onto the belt.

4. Gently flex the fingers around
   the plain end of the belt.

4. Grasp the end of the belt.

5. Gently place your hand
   over the client's hand, so that
   it is grasping the belt, and
   move the belt to the first loop
   on the pants, pointing to the
   loop at the same time.

5. Lift the belt into the
   position of the first loop.

Ordinarily, it will not be necessary to specify steps for both worker and
client. However, it is important that the same sequence of events occur in
each training session. For this reason, workers who are learning this type of
training may well wish to use such a detailed plan until intimately familiar
with the method. For those who wish to implement training programs, a
large number of complete task analyses are available commercially from
Marc Gold & Associates (see Appendix). Many of these are quite appropriate for the needs of APB clients with little modification.

Sometimes special equipment becomes a necessary adjunct to the
training process. Special utensils for eating and for assistance in dressing,
for example, are available from several companies, some of which are listed
in the Appendix. In addition, occupational and physical therapists are often
excellent sources of ideas for adaptive equipment and techniques, and for
modifying existing materials for use in teaching various skills. Following is
a list of simple modifications to readily available devices which may be of
value in training, particularly with the physically disabled APB client:

Independent Eating

1. Place a wet wash cloth under dishes to keep them from
   sliding.
2. Press plates, saucers, and bowls into modeling clay stuck on
   to the table to keep them steady.
3. Put a pencil clip on a straw and hook it to a drinking glass,
   to hold straw in place.
4. Build up handles of eating utensils with clay, tape or foam
   for easier gripping.

Dressing

1. Put leather or ribbon tabs on zippers for easier gripping.
2. Attach pieces of velcro to clothing and to elastic bands which can be worn on client's hands for assistance with grasping and pulling on clothing.

Personal Hygiene

1. Make a washcloth mitten.
2. Make elastic washcloth bands so that they can be slipped around the client's hands.
3. Attach a sponge to a rod or dowel for washing hard to reach parts of the body.
4. Build up the toothbrush grip with tape or foam rubber, or stick a small rubber ball on the end of handle.
5. Place a wide band of elastic around a bar of soap for easier gripping or so that the client's hand can be slipped under the elastic.

When training a skill which involves the use of equipment (e.g., glass, toothbrush, toothpaste) it is often helpful to arrange it on the shelf in the order in which it will be used. As with the sequence of steps in other manual training, the order should never be changed during training. Adaptive devices such as those discussed above can be quite helpful, but should not be used unless necessary, since they draw attention to the clients deviance and may lend support to negative attributional self-statements.

It will be noted that the task analysis material presented here includes no verbal cues or reinforcement. When training manual skills, it is important that the client attend to the task at hand; verbal instructions and remarks may compete with more relevant stimuli, to the detriment of learning.

A great deal has been written about the use of multisensory cues in prosthetic environments. Inasmuch as these cues are non-competing, the rationale for their use holds up. For example, the use of large numerals and color coding to designate patient rooms is likely to be more successful in orienting residents to place than would either method alone, since either cue, or both, can be salient. The resident has a choice—a self-determination—that allows selective attention to the most relevant cue.

There seems to be a tendency to assume that if multisensory stumuli are useful in this situation, they must also work best for other problems. The problem with verbal instructions or cues is that they are typically erratic, unstandardized and tend to "lag" behind actual performance. If timing is not precisely contiguous to the behavior, the client may have already proceeded to the next step, and the cue represents non-relevant information, or interference. With most APB clients, manual cues alone seem most efficient in training ADL skills, with only word reinforcement (e.g., "OK") when a step is accomplished correctly, or none at all if the trainer is comfortable with this approach. Gold's approach of using the phrase "Try another way" to correct a client who is making a mistake may also be helpful as an alternative to manual correction. The point is simply that all verbal communication, once training is underway, should be kept to a minimum, using only cues that are demonstrably efficacious in improving task learning.

This is not to imply that spoken communication has no place in training. The client has a right to know what is happening, so that he or she can decide whether to participate, and under what conditions. Regardless of the client's supposed intellectual deficits, this should be undertaken before any training is done. That is as far as verbal communication need go, however.

A final important element of this form of training is the need for systematic assessment of training progress. If independent dressing is the goal, it is helpful to maintain a chart on which the successful completion of steps can be recorded, along with whether the client was able to perform it alone, in what setting, at what time of day, and with which trainer. This gives invaluable information regarding the training process itself (such as steps that are especially difficult and perhaps too complex) and situational variables (e.g., better performance in the morning or with a particular trainer) that may suggest helpful changes in the training procedure. A recording form such as the sample which follows this chapter can be modified as necessary to adequately assess client progress during training.

Far from being a mechanistic, over-standardized procedure, the general principles and techniques suggested in this chapter find application in a most individualized fashion. Every client enters training with different skills, abilities, and aspirations. Due to the very nature of the APB syndrome, however, there is very little direct feedback to the trainer from the client, and even using powerful training procedures progress will often be slow. Systematic progress assessment is therefore essential, and should be looked upon as a work saver, not an additional chore for overworked staff.

SUMMARY

We have attempted to define an underserved population of institutionalized elderly, named after its most visible and salient single characteristic: the apparent absence of purposeful behavior. Regardless of precipitating medical and/or psychiatric events that lead to institutional care, a major reason that such persons remain is that their performance of self-care or self-enhancing competencies is so impaired that total nursing care is required. It is

Sample Recording Form

Skill: Putting on a belt

Terminal Objective: Each day, after putting on his socks, underwear, shirt and
pants, client will take his belt from the closet and put it on,
correctly buckling it.

Tasks: 1. Extend the fingers on the dominant hand.
2. Move the hand over the plain end of the belt.
3. Lower the hand onto the belt.
4. Grasp the plain end of the belt.
5. Lift the belt end to the first loop position.

Client: _____

Entering Skills:_____

Date & Time	Trainer's Name	1	2	Tasks 3	4	5	Comments

Ratings: 1 = client completed task unassisted
2 = client needed partial assistance
3 = client needed total assistance

hypothesized that, in addition to problems the client brings to the hospital,
there are certain ubiquitous characteristics of the health care setting itself
that contribute to the severity of the client's impairment.

Three issues relating to the dearth of treatment or training programs
for APB clients were identified. First, staff attitudes are often negativistic,

based upon perception of the client as permanently and totally disabled, with the locus of disability entirely within the client. This contributes to further dependency-producing treatment practices and thus, perpetuates the low functional level of APB clients. A second issue concerns the selection of skills to be taught, particularly in view of potential conflicts between staff wishes and client motivation (e.g., desire to learn "fun" or recreational skills rather than ADL). A list of desirable self-care and recreational skills was provided, along with a discussion of skill selection procedures. The final issue is the development of an appropriate training technology. Drawing on attributional concepts as well as behavioral techniques from the field of mental retardation, one possible training "package" was suggested. Principal components include task analysis procedures and reinforcement or feedback considerations that aid performance and should not contribute to clients' negative self-image.

With due recognition that this approach is no panacea, that the issues discussed are not inclusive, and that the techniques require systematic empirical validation on the APB populace, we nonetheless believe that this represents a framework on which to build therapeutic interventions for this group of impaired elderly.

Appendix

Suppliers of Equipment and Training Aids

Cleo Living Aids
3957 Mayfield Road
Cleveland, Ohio 44121

Marc Gold & Associates
P.O. Box 5100
Austin, Texas 78763

Fred Sammons, Inc.
Box 32
Brookfield, Illinois 60513

North American Recreation
Convertibles
P.O. Box 668
Westport, Connecticut 06880

G. E. Miller, Inc.
484 South Broadway
Yonkers, New York 10705

Ortho-Kinetics, Inc.
P.O. Box 463
Waukesha, Wisconsin 53136

J. A. Preston Corp.
71 Fifth Avenue
New York, New York 10003

Skill Development Equipment
P.O. Box 6497
Anaheim, California 92806

References

Azrin, N. H., Sneed, J. R., & Foxx, R. M. Dry bed: A rapid method of eliminating bedwetting (enuresis) of the retarded. *Mental Retardation*, 1973, *2:* 9-13

Botwinick, J. *Aging and behavior* (2nd Ed.). New York: Springer Publishing Co., 1978.

Gold, M. *Try another way: training manual.* Champaign, Ill.: Institute for Child Behavior and Development, University of Illinios at Urbana-Champaign, 1975.

Richards, W. S., & Thorpe, G. L. Behavioral approaches to the problems of later life. In M. Storandt, I. D. Siegler, & M. F. Elias (eds.), *The clinical psychology of aging.* New York: Plenum Press, 1978.

Weiner, B. Achievement motivation as conceptualized by an attribution theorist. In B. Weiner (ed.), *Achievement motivation and attribution theory.* Morristown, N.J.: General Learning Press, 1974.

Weiner, B., Frieze, I., Kukla, A., Reed, L., Rest, S., & Rosenbaum, R. M. Perceiving the causes of success and failure. In E. E. Jones, D. E. Kanouse, H. H. Kelly, R. E. Nisbett, S. Valins, & B. Weiner (eds.), *Perceiving the causes of behavior.* Morristown, N.J.: General Learning Press, 1972.

Williams, W., Brown, L., & Certo, N. Basic components of instructional programs. In R. M. Anderson and J. G. Greer (eds.), *Educating the severely and profoundly retarded.* Baltimore: University Park Press, 1976.

5
Facilitating a Better Reality: A Treatment Approach for the Confused and Disoriented

Christine A. Lewis

AN ORIENTATION TO REALITY ORIENTATION

Aging is a dynamic concept that may be considered from several frames of reference. Medically, it is described as structural change that occurs over time, is not caused by disease or accident, and eventually increases the probability of death. Sociologists stress the adaptational and social assistance needs of elderly citizens confronted with altered family, occupational, and social roles. The arbitrary designation of an aged person as someone sixty-five years of age or older reflects this perspective as it corresponds with the former manditory retirement age. Gerontological psychologists emphasize the cognitive and emotional concomitants of normal or disease-related physiological change, environmental modification, and disrupted interpersonal relationships. Popularly, growing older is resisted or relished depending on one's attitudes toward personal senescence. Aging is certainly a process of physical and social change that forces adaptations, a mental and emotional response to life's events, and a reaction to preconceived notions or images. This description could apply to any phase of the human lifespan except for the anticipations of disability, senility, institutionalization and imminent death which lend it a grimmer character.

The effects of aging are not so easily predicted, however, for they vary widely within the general population and between individuals of identical ages. It is not thoroughly understood how or why the biological changes associated with growing older occur but it has become generally accepted that one's habitual health care, lifestyle, and mental outlook prior to reaching chronological old age can effect physical aging. It is in the arena of construction health practices and preventative medicine that aging may begin to yield some of its unassailable symptoms.

Presently acknowledged facts of aging are discussed by Palmore (1977) who cited several sources to document various physical, psychological, and socioeconomic aspects of growing old. Many are pertinent to later discussion. The acuity of hearing, vision, touch, taste, and smell is reported to diminish with advancing age. Lung capacity and physical strength have been found to decline with the latter ranging between a 15% and 48% reduction compared to young adults. Reaction time has been studied in numerous ways and has consistently evidenced slackening in older people. Learning of new material or skills is described as slower and more dependent on repetition for aged persons but is then similar to learning in younger people. Concluding a review of incidence data, Dr. Palmore stated, "all the evidence indicates that there are less than 10% of the aged who are disoriented or demented." Diminished long-term memory capacity was found in less than 20% of the older population. Further evidence indicated little or no decline in short-term memory storage capacity as measured by digit span tests. Palmore also reported that: (a) 80% of the aged population remains sufficiently healthy to pursue normal activities, (b) 4.8% of the citizens over sixty-five years old are institutionalized, and (c) 9.2% of those seventy-five years of age or older are residents of long-term care facilities. To summarize, aging does result in diminishments of mental and physical abilities but it neither incapacitates the majority of elderly adults nor dictates a lockstep into institutional care. This premise of aging as a multifarious, idiosyncratic, and noncrippling process has significance for those who experience problematic mental deterioration.

Faulty Assumptions About Mental Impairment

It's normal to be senile. One attitude being challenged is the perfunctory dismissal of symptoms to "old age." Medical examination has been traditionally vital since numerous diseases and physical traumas have presented symptoms that include, among others, confusion, disorientation and faulty memory. Cape (1978) stated these symptoms, especially if acute, constitute a medical emergency requiring prompt treatment. Careful exploration is also called for in three additional realms, psychological reaction, sensory deprivation, and environmental incompatibility. Several authors (Barnes 1974; Jahraus 1974; Lee 1976a; Citrin and Dixon 1977; Voelkel 1978) have maintained that psychological reactions may exacerbate or mimic symptoms of debility thought to have an organic etiology. Among the most frequent aspects discussed are (a) the withdrawal, apathy, and depression associated with both social isolation and the death of loved ones or friends; (b) the bewilderment and anxiety observed when events threaten self-esteem and feeling of security; (c) identity disturbances arising from the loss of autonomy and important social roles; and (d) the helplessness learned in environments that foster dependency through low expectations and overprotectiveness. Sensory deprivation, broadly considered a lack of activity and/or deterioration of the sense organs, may be a root cause of behavior described as confused, especially if recent memory is impaired (Woods and Britton 1977). Appropriate behavioral responses to the environment are seen as dependent on accurate perceptions which in turn create a cognitive representation of reality on which actions are premised. Sparse, faulty, or forgotten perceptions make it difficult to maintain an adequate idea of the environment and may thus lead to confused behavior. Cape (1978) mentioned a final precipitating factor, environmental incompatability. He cited several aspects of modern living such as the need to travel long distances to obtain services and the fast pace of daily events which may strain the elderly individual to the limits of his or her coping abilities. Should demands become intolerable, confusion may be among the earliest symptoms observed. Pragmatically, variables within these four areas are likely to interact with one another and with the normal biological changes of advancing age. An etiological determination is thus complex but, when met, establishes the foundation on which to anticipate a patient's potential for recovery.

There's little hope for improvement. Another common presumption is that symptoms of mental impairment in an aged person are chronic, i.e., irreversible. While critical of various methodological flaws in current studies, Woods and Britton (1977) concluded, "There is...an increasing body of evidence that a sizable investment of therapeutic endeavor may produce improvement [and] deterioration need not be continuous and inevitable." Isler (1975) described an eclectic approach to geriatric care in which 100 patients admitted for depression, confusion, agitation, or organic brain syndrome were involved. She stated, "more than half showed significant response" to the care provided and were discharged. Katz (1976) conducted an observational study of 108 patients living in an extended care facility. The staff intuitively ranked the residents as mildly, moderately, or severely confused. All subjects participated in "multimodal group interactive therapy" for eighteen months. A final ranking was obtained. Improvement was reported in 44% of the participants with 23% remaining stable, 15% worsening and 18% transferring before the program ended. Both Cape (1978) and Wertz (1979) distinguished between medically precipitated confusion and dementia. They agreed that etiology prognosticates recovery from confusion whereas age is an additional factor to consider with dementia. Prognostic demographic factors were not mentioned. Early identification and prompt intervention were urged as each author maintained that improvements were most likely under these circumstances.

Although positive behavioral changes are reported, the issue of whether or not they constitute a real difference, i.e. enable a person to reacquire a recognizable degree of independence and/or emotional well being, is pivotal. Implied is the necessity for behavioral assessment and periodic reappraisal during treatment phases. This constitutes a major goal to be satisfied if more specific prognostic indicators and justifiable intervention strategies are desirable.

The diagnosis should dictate treatment. A final assumption being criticized is that treatment paradigms are prescriptive to diagnosis. One can recognize this tenet in operation in a variety of ways. A particular diagnosis may be so general as to mask the severity and variability of symptoms it subsumes, i.e. chronic organic brain syndrome, and yet be selected to describe individuals for whom a certain program is recommended. This can conceivably result in ineffectual pairing of patients with a form of intervention or lead to premature or prolonged involvement of patients with a program that has its greatest value only during certain phases of rehabilitation. Another problem of permitting a diagnosis to determine treatment arises when coexisting diagnoses are present. Should one overshadow others, the neglect of important factors is risked which could reduce the benefits to be derived from therapeutic efforts. For example, a person manifesting confusion secondary to head trauma but also having a significant sensori-neural hearing impairment may participate in a group without the compensations of preferential seating, good lighting, and a functioning hearing aid. Conflict can also exist when one diagnosis might logically assume primacy over others. A terminal cancer patient who behaves in a confused manner might best be served through a Hospice program rather than in a reality orientation program even though the latter could contain some supportive techniques. A further difficulty is encountered when a symptom is shared by more than one diagnostic category. A potentially helpful treatment approach may be avoided because a patient differs from others in his classification. At times this is attributable to a terminological quandary rather than a genuine behavioral difference.

Diagnosis is certainly as essential as establishing the etiology of signs and symptoms. By organizing observations and data into a recognizable pattern and assigning a label to it, communication between care-givers is eased and exceptions or complications to an anticipated pattern are highlighted. The time required for a detailed behavioral and medical diagnosis is rewarded by more efficient and pertinent program delivery. The above pitfalls of planning from a diagnosis can be minimized by making each label specific, by reaching a consensus among members of a multidisciplinary staff on the denotative meaning of the labels used, and by maintaining a perspective that appreciates the unique gestalt of each patient. A staff terminology guide can be useful. The goals are a detailed approach for eliminating, reversing, or counteracting the causes and effects of mental deterioration and an optimal placement plan that best complies with a patient's needs and resources.

Historical Foundation of Reality Orientation

Thoughout the past two decades, the aging person with failing mental skills and the custodial nature of the care s/he has typically received have been reconsidered. The period has been seminal to the development of various psychotherapeutic approaches geared specifically to elderly patients. Woods and Britton (1977) reviewed techniques reported to be effective and found them to have several shared features. Programs were intensive in order to maximize opportunities of learning to occur. Active patient participation was characteristic since behavior to be shaped or reinforced had to first be elicited. Adequate and relevant consequences that acknowledged accomplishments were used to build and sustain motivation. Lastly, staff education and sensitization was integrated to promote constructive attitudes toward geriatric care.

Reality Orientation (RO) was among the procedures considered effective. It is a multifaceted stimulation approach designed for use with individuals exhibiting confusion and/or disorientation. It is founded on four premises: (a) physiological changes only partially account for the symptoms of confusion or disorientation, (b) without therapeutic intervention, individuals manifesting these symptoms will progressively deteriorate in their abilities to carry out daily living activities, (c) direct, active, and positive strategies have remedial and preventative effects and serve to accentuate behavioral assets necessary for independence, and (d) RO procedures and techniques are relevant to a broad range of patients who vary etiologically and diagnostically.

Dr. James C. Folsom (1968), the originator of RO, detailed its evolution from an earlier form entitled "aide-centered activity" which was introduced in 1958 at the Veterans Administration Hospital in Topeka, Kansas. Fifty patients housed on a long-term care ward were engaged in group activities devised and carried out by nursing assistants. Rehabilitation therapists supervised until assistants became skilled enough to assume the initiative. Team conferences were conducted routinely to include the aides. The benefits cited were increased physical independence of patients, improved socialization between patient members, decreased injury and intercurrent infections among patients, and improved staff morale as reflected by a decrease of lost-time accidents, reduced use of sick leave, and fewer requests for reassignment.

The next phase began in 1961 at the Mental Health Institute in Mt. Pleasant, Iowa, where Dr. Folsom was serving as clinical director. A staff physician expressed concern that only 3% of the geriatric patients were improving sufficiently to be returned to their former lifestyle. It was decided to conduct a pilot program incorporating the philosophies of the Topeka project and introducing techniques of attitude therapy. Patients were accepted into the program if they were new admissions over sixty-five years old, ambulatory, and "mentally ill," regardless of severity. After six months, the multidisciplinary staff established a set of guidelines for helping confused patients reorient themselves. These tenets became the essential elements of what was termed "reality orientation." The maintenance of family contact was also emphasized. At the conclusion of the one-year project, 5% of the participating patients were able to return to their prehospital setting.

In 1965, Dr. Folsom continued his efforts at the Veterans Administration Hospital in Tuscaloosa, Alabama, with "psychiatric medically infirm patients." Added elements included a twenty-four-hour emphasis on treatment, structured orientation classes, and environmental props. Within a one-year period, sixty-four patients had been assigned to the program. Outplacement was achieved by 14% of the participants, 12.5% remained hospitalized with privileges increased, and 45% continued active in the program. An attrition of 28.5% was attributed to patient deaths, illness, or uncooperativeness. After four and one-half years, the project had involved 227 patients of whom 20% completed classes but remained at the facility and 20% had been discharged (Stephens 1969). Encouraged by these results, the institution's staff began its ongoing, comprehensive Reality Orientation Training Program. During the forty-hour workshops, caregivers are trained to apply the principles and techniques developed in the five distinct areas constituting a complete RO program: twenty-four-hour intervention, environmental support, classroom activity, behavioral management, and family education.

Research Endeavors

A total approach. The studies conducted to ascertain the effects of intervention following the RO paradigm need to be grouped according to the actual elements implemented in the research design. One group of investigations incorporates at least three of the five basic features, i.e. twenty-four-hour intervention, environmental support, and classroom activity. Letcher, Peterson, and Scarbrough (1974) reported on a post hoc analysis of 125 patient records accumulated over five years. Organic brain syndrome secondary to cerebral arteriosclerosis was the primary diagnosis for 80% of the cases. An additional 15% had a diagnosis of cerebral vascular accident. The mean age of the patients was 82.8 years. Improvement was determined by comparing nursing-care level at intake with that at discharge. Overall, 32% of the patients improved and 68% remained stable. An analysis of demographic characteristics evidenced no significant trends. The rate of improvement was highest for patients who had participated for at least 18 months and who were initially more self-sufficient.

Harris and Ivory (1976) selected two groups of twenty-nine women each from a state hospital setting. Subjects were matched for age and diagnosis. Syphilis, organic brain syndrome, and mental deficiency were the most frequent diagnostic categories. The average length of hospitalization exceeded twenty years for both groups. The experimental group was provided with RO in addition to the typical ward routine followed by the control group. A scale rating twenty-six behaviors was completed by two aides for each patient prior to the five-month experimental period and at its conclusion. There were no significant differences between groups on pretest data. Only verbal orientation behaviors improved significantly in the experimental group by the end of the study. In 1977, Citrin and Dixon also reported a significant improvement of verbal orientation for their experimental group of twelve elderly patients who averaged eighty-four years of age and exhibited "moderate confusion." These subjects remained comparable to the thirteen control subjects in activities of daily living when the study was concluded after seven weeks.

Classroom investigations. A second set of studies incorporates frequent classes using an environmental prop but do not report following a plan for twenty-four-hour intervention. One early project (Barnes 1974) employed a twenty-three-item questionnaire to screen patients for classes and to measure progress. Twelve patients who exhibited moderate to severe confusion, disorientation, or memory loss were enrolled. Six subjects having a mean age of eighty-one years actually completed the six-week program in which half-hour classes were conducted six days a week. Statistically significant changes were not obtained except for a decline in scores between post-test scores and data obtained one week later.

Holden and Sinebruchow (1978) reported on both an uncontrolled pilot project and a controlled study in which patients varied etiologically (depression, Parkinson's disease and stroke) and were medically stable, continent, and nonviolent. The pilot project involved fourteen subjects with a mean age of eighty years and an average length of institutionalization of 1.75 years. One-hour orientation classes were held five or six times a week for three months. Although statistical analysis of pre-and post-test data revealed no significant gains, these researchers were encouraged by the fact that five patients could be discharged and six patients had improved their initial scores. The controlled study drew patients from two different facilities. Subjects had similar diagnostic and behavioral characteristics to their first sample. The experimental group of sixteen subjects averaged seventy-seven years of age and 1.4 years of institutionalization. The sixteen control subjects were slightly older, an average of 79.9 years, and had been in the nursing home longer, a mean of 1.96 years. The Stockton Geriatric Rating Scale and the Clifton Assessment Schedule were administered prior to commencing daily, one-hour classes and therafter at intervals of two, six, and twelve weeks. Statistical significance was not reached. The experimental group had more discharges and more patients improving over their initial test performance. Likewise, Hogstel (1979) conducted a controlled study with forty geriatric patients. Half of the subjects participated in classroom activities five times a week for a total of three weeks but did not evidence statistically significant gains on an eighteen-item verbal orientation questionnaire.

Another study (Cornbleth & Cornbleth 1979) enrolled twenty-two patients in five half-hour sessions a week after it had been determined that degree of confusion manifested by patients was within a moderate to severe range. All subjects had a diagnosis of organic brain syndrome. The mean age and length of hospitalization were seventy-five years and 5.34 years, respectively. A thirty-item verbal orientation questionnaire and an eighty-five-item behavioral checklist were administered by nursing personnel prior to initiating classes and three months later when the program ended. The authors concluded that the significant improvement derived statistically from both scales was evidence for reality orientation's effectiveness.

Comparative studies. Other researchers have compared orientation classes to other forms of intervention. Brook, Degun, and Mather (1975) hypothesized that environmental enrichment alone could benefit patients in geriatric wards and that active involvement with a therapist would promote even greater gains.They accepted eighteen demented patients as subjects after it was determined that they were nonviolent, continent, ambulatory, intact sensorily, and not excessively sedated. Their average age was seventy-three years and they had been hospitalized for an average of 1.9 years. Computer analysis clustered subjects according to severity from scores obtained on a rating scale devised by the authors. Patients were randomly assigned to either the control group which experienced a change in enviornment only or the experimental group which participated in RO classes in the enriched environment. The rating scale was readministered every two weeks for a period of sixteen weeks. Data analysis supported the study's hypotheses with both groups improving the first two weeks and only the experimental group maintaining or improving upon the initial gains by the end of the study. Moderately to mildly impaired patients responded best to orientation activities.

In 1978, McDonald and Settin reported on a comparison between a reality orientation group, a sheltered workshop group, and an assessment-only control group. Their thirty subjects were selected on the basis of having adequate vision, hearing, and speech, mobility of one arm, and a willingness to participate. Confusion was not a criterion. Group assignment was random with fifty-minute sessions held for all but the control subjects. Classes met three times a week for five weeks. Pre- and post-test measures were obtained using the Life Satisfaction Index, Nurses' Observation Scale for Inpatient Evaluation, and Behavior Mapping Index. The sheltered workshop group evidenced significant gains on the Life Satisfaction Index and on ratings for being "socially interested" compared to the other groups.

Voelkel (1978) studied twenty patients for six weeks. They had been randomly assigned to either a reality orientation class or to a resocialization group after initial screening for moderate to severe confusion. Pfeiffer's Short Portable Mental Status Questionnaire was used for this purpose and for assessing improvement. Citing the t-test results but not reporting the data, she stated that the resocialization group, which had higher initial scores, improved significantly over the reality orientation group. In a similar vein, Woods (1979) compared three groups of six patients each. They had been selected on the basis of age, mental incapacity, and ability to complete the psychological tests chosen for the study, i.e. Wechsler Memory Scale, Memory and Information Test, Clifton Assessment Schedule, and a modification of the Crichton Rating Scale. Patients were randomly assigned to an orientation group, a socialization group, or an assessment-only control group. Assessments were repeated after three, nine and twenty weeks of sessions which were held for thirty minutes a day, five days a week. All groups were initially comparable with respect to age and test performance. Except for performance on the rating scale for which no treatment effect was apparent, the group participating in reality orientation classes was statistically superior to the other two groups. Improvements were significant as early as three weeks and were maintained throughout the remaining weeks of the study. An exception was the performance levels of the Wechsler which were not significantly better until the ninth week but were then maintained.

Case study. A series of three case studies (Green, Nicol, and Jamieson 1979) sought to assess the effects of training using orientation questions only. Dr. Green et al., reported data on three female, demented patients seen individually for thirty-minute sessions in a day hospital. They used an ABAB design in which either correct answers only were acknowledged (condition A) or correct answers were given if a patient made an error or no response (condition B). On the basis of this format, they concluded that orientation could be improved by this simple procedure and that improvement was neither a stimulation effect nor stereotyped response. Generalization occurred to behavior dependent on orientation but not to social behavior. The patient with moderate dementia responded best in terms of generalization and maintenance of gains.

Summary. Comparison between studies is made difficult by the varied and/or unspecified etiological and diagnostic information on subjects, the range, quantity, and quality of assessment procedures used, and the disparity between investigators' application of reality orientation either in the features included or in the duration of the projects. As a total approach, it appears to effect positive and significant changes in verbal orientation in a fairly brief time. The predominant image in terms of patient self-sufficiency is one of stability although some patients did improve given a lengthier time frame. When only classroom activities were introduced, statistically significant gains were not found except in one careful but un-controlled study. Compared to environmental enrichment or socialization, reality orientation groups did evidence greater benefits to confused patients. When confusion was not a defining characteristic of a group, another type of intervention appeared more appropriate. Individualized treatment emphasizing orientation may hold promise as well. Several investigators suggested that patients exhibiting moderate incapacity responded the best to reorientation efforts.

THE STRUCTURE OF A REALITY ORIENTATION PROGRAM

Important Implications

The definition of RO as a stimulation technique for confused and/or disoriented individuals contains several implications. Stimulation must be adequate in order for the approach to be valid. All avenues of input—sight, sound, scent, taste and touch—hold potential for exploitation. Recalling that diminishment of sensation is a normal consequence of aging and that other factors can affect sensory acuity, variables such as the frequency, duration, and variety of stimulation, the size, intensity, and distinctiveness of stimulus materials, and the relevance of information to be gained require careful consideration. Secondly, RO's appropriate application is with con-fused and/or disoriented patients. It has a symptomatic focus; however, im-plied is the need for assessment. Staff should determine the existence and severity of these symptoms, establish their etiology, specify the broader diagnostic category to which these symptoms belong, and note the presence of any complicating conditions. In other words, every attempt should be made to assure that this intervention strategy corresponds to a patient's needs.

Perhaps not immediately apparent is the fact that RO techniques are used as a part of a total rehabilitation plan. A multidisciplinary team is con-sidered vital. Phillips (1973) went to the extent of stating that "Reality Orientation can be effective only when a total team approach is used." Under optimal conditions, the team is composed of each staff person who routinely has contact with the patient. This could include a dietician, chaplin, and orderly along with the primary care physician, psychologist, nurse, social worker, and physical rehabilitation specialists. One often overlooked member of a team in some settings, but not in an RO program, is the patient. S/he is encouraged to participate in team discussions and is kept informed about pertinent decisions even when it is not certain s/he will fully comprehend. Different settings will certainly vary in terms of the personnel resources available to them. The essential point to retain is that without a coordinated and cooperating staff to assess, develop, implement and revise a course of action, rehabilitative efforts risk fragmentation and disjuncture. The greater the number of people interacting with a patient, the more likely the patient's confusion or disorientation will be aggrevated should staff coordination be absent.

Given its historical roots and the variety of guises it has been given in the research literature, Reality Orientation can be appreciated for its versatility. It is offered as a form of intervention for a broad range of etiologically and diagnostically disparate patients. The aims of the program will vary. It may be introduced during acute phases when prevention is its main purpose. RO is employed with preventative, remedial, and maintenance intents when the precipitating conditions or their effects are chronic. It functions as support for patients whose diseases are degenerative. Further, flexibility is found in the settings in which RO may be efficacious: acute care units (Burnside 1977), transition units (Cornbleth and Cornbleth 1979), nursing homes (Phillips 1973), day hospitals (Greene et al., 1979) and mental hospitals (Harris and Ivory 1976). Finally, it can be practiced by any trained individual and entail different combinations of features. It is the adherence to specific guidelines that is the one characteristic by which RO is understood as a constant amid diversity.

General Guidelines

Several broad guidelines were established early in the development of Reality Orientation (Folsom 1968). These tenets are fundamental to the reorientation of confused or disoriented patients irregardless of how one specifically implements a program. Since their inception, Hackley (1973) and Scarbrough (1974) have reiterated them and several program descriptions encompassed them throughout the discussions (AHA 1973; Drummond, Kirchhoff, and Scarbrough 1978; Hefferin and Hunter 1977; Lee 1976 a and b; Phillips 1973; Stephens 1969; Taulbee 1973). Although summarized and explained here from a staff perspective, these same guidelines can be followed by family members or anyone else interacting with a confused or disoriented individual.

1. The environment is calm, minimally distracting, and characterized by predictability in staff and routine. The aim is to create an atmosphere in which a patient can find security through familiarity and reassurance

through predictability. Because structuring events and responding to sudden changes can pose problems for the patient, it is the staff's responsibility to provide and follow a set routine, to highlight the repetitive aspects of each day, to seek means of eliminating distractions, to anticipate and announce nonroutine events, to stabilize staffing patterns, and to react calmly to unexpected events.

2. Verbal communication from staff members to patients is straightforward, unambiguous, distinct, and supplemented by demonstration, assistance, or guidance when needed. The purpose is to assist patients to restructure their world through socialization. The emphasis is placed on the present for which patients have a point of reference. The staff should attempt to bring each interaction to a logical conclusion and to acknowledge appropriate statements from patients.

3. Information about time, person, place, and expectations is repeated frequently throughout the day. The rationale for repetition is to circumvent or compensate for such common difficulties as faulty recall, shortened attention span, distractability, and inaccurate associations and to thereby maximize the likelihood of information being received and retained. Such information can be provided by the staff in varied ways. This purposeful redundancy usually constitutes a challenge for a staff to maintain until its benefits in reorienting patients is observed.

4. Confused or disoriented behavior in either a patient's speech or actions is immediately interrupted and corrected. The purpose of this practice is twofold: to break the vicious cycle of one inappropriate behavior leading to another and to reestablish self-perception and self-control. Error feedback and correction is one means by which inappropriate behavior is underscored and appropriate alternatives are provided.

5. The staff practices restraint from hurrying a patient to respond and from assisting a patient when capability exists. The expectation from this guideline is that a staff will sensitize itself to the misguided means by which helplessness is taught, will eliminate those practices that foster dependency, and will encourage high degrees of self-sufficiency in patients. Such changes as eliminating the convenience of a wheelchair when a patient can walk, albeit slowly, to appointments, allocating more time for grooming before meals, or establishing a bladder retraining schedule in lieu of cathedarization would be in keeping with this guideline.

6. The staff reflects an attitude toward patients that is respectfully firm, sincere, polite, and adult. In essence, this is responding to the daily demands of patient care from an empathetic yet professional base. Through positive attitudes, a staff can create an atmosphere conducive to reestablishing and maintaining a patient's self-esteem.

7. Techniques are applied consistently. The intent is to intensify the effects of intervention in promoting reorientation and self-sufficiency by assuring its presence from day-to-day, setting-to-setting, and person-to-person. It is achieved through coordination, cooperation, and careful communication between all persons relating to the patient.

Key Features of a Complete Reality Orientation Program

Twenty-four Hour RO. Premised on a view that every utterance constitutes an intervention, this aspect of the program provides orienting information whenever the patient is awake. It is a style of verbal interaction that repeatedly emphasizes information about person, place, time, ongoing activity, and behavioral expectation. It typically occurs in a one-to-one exchange either as a simultaneous adjunct to an activity, as a corrective measure during an episode of confusion or disorientation, or as a preventative technique when confused or disoriented behavior is anticipated. Burnside (1977) pointed out five situations when "reality testing must be considered. . . :immediately following electro-shock treatment, during the stage from sleep to wakefulness, during acute confusional states. . . .during reactions from drugs or alcohol, [and] during illusions." She recommended that personnel (a) listen purposefully in order to determine what elements of reality are mutually perceived and which ones are being misinterpreted, (b) explain the unfamiliar, (c) have accurate information before contradicting a patient's statement, (d) avoid arguments over differing conceptions, and (e) attempt to allay fears and apprehensions.

Before starting twenty-four hour RO, it should be appreciated that, although simple, this type of communication does not develop spontaneously. Anyone who would be routinely interacting with the patient, including family members, visitors, or volunteers, needs both training and practical experience before its delivery is natural and consistent. Once training is accomplished, they should be cautioned against the common misapplication of narrowing communication with patients to a robot-like presentation of orienting information only. This violates the intent of RO by neglecting a patient's individuality and social needs. One can eliminate its occurrence by first allowing sufficient time for patients to respond so they can demonstrate some facet of their knowledge and, secondly, by engaging patients in other conversation after the necessary orienting topics have been presented. If patients do not respond, orienting facts should still be stated in as conversational a manner as possible.

A particularly sensitive area in twenty-four hour RO is introducing painful aspects of reality, e.g., the fact of a spouse's death. Taulbee (1973) stated, "truth will be accepted if it is explained simply and slowly by a trusted, understanding person. It may aid the patient's understanding if events leading up to the fact are related to him. Abruptness is traumatic and often leads to refusal to accept reality." Generally, a staff should neither avoid relating painful facts nor support a patient's confusion or denial about such facts. When doubt exists about how to convey potentially upsetting information, expert advice can be obtained either through a multidisciplinary team conference or consultation procedures.

The following examples illustrate the types of exchanges one might observe in a setting practicing twenty-four hour RO: when carrying out a routine activity,

> Good morning, Mr. Swartz (a polite greeting giving time and person information). My name is Mary Lee (person). I am your nurse (person) on the day shift (time). It is 9:00 Monday morning (time). I am in your room (place) to take your blood pressure (ongoing activity). Please hold out your right arm (behavioral expectation). Did you like your breakfast this morning (general conversation)?

when correcting an episode of disorientation,

> "Mr. Swartz (person), it's 2:00 in the morning (time) You are sup-posed to be sleeping (behavioral expection) in your room (place)," "No, I'm changing my clothes and going swimming." Patient starts for the shower room. The nurse remembers the patient had routinely swum laps at the YMCA. "Yes, this shower room looks like a locker room (acknowleges correct aspect of perception) but this is not the YMCA. This is the Hillside Nursing Home (corrects misperception). I'm Sue Bennett (person), your night nurse (time/person). It's very early in the morning (time) and you should be sleeping (behavioral ex-pectation). Did something wake you?" "No...yes. I need the bathroom." "I'll show you where your bathroom is (ongoing activity). Here is your bathroom (place)."

and when anticipating a potentially confusing moment.

> Mr. Swartz (person), it's time to wake up (time). Good morning (time), Mr. Swartz (person), please wake up now (behavioral expecta-tion). It's 7:30 Tuesday morning (time). I'm Mary Lee, your day nurse (person) here at Hillside Nursing Home (place). Please sit up (behavioral expectation), Mr. Swarz (person). Thank you (compliance acknowledged). I'm here to help you get ready for breakfast (ongoing activity). Here are your slippers and bathrobe to put on (behavioral expectation).

When engaging in twenty-four hour RO as exemplified, the aim is to con-sistently provide information that patients need for self-orientation. Once they are able to do so, the content needs not be specific. If a patient greets a staff member by name, there would be no necessity for that person to give his or her name. Questions may be asked to ascertain if a patient knows facts before they are stated. Finally, environmental cues helpful to consistently provide information that patients need for orientation can be referred to and associated with conversational content.

Environmental RO. Supplementing and complementing twenty-four-hour RO are various environmental props which serve as reminders of person, place, time, and activities. One popular prop is the RO board. It has an announcement format with interchangeable, easy-to-read words to complete each section. The name of the facility and its city and state locations are at the top. Succeeding lines read: Today is_____, The date is_____, The weather is_____, The next holiday is_____, The next meal is_____. The board can be altered to fit the requirements in any particular setting. Boards are displayed prominantly in several areas where patients tend to congregate. Anyone can refer to the prop during conversations with patients and can encourage its use as a resource. Other traditional props are clocks with large numbers that are mounted low on walls for easy visibility, and calendars.

Other environmental alterations are suggested to accommodate confused or disoriented patients. Color-coded doors and hallways, large room numbers, pictographic signs, and simplified maps of the facility can help patients locate places more easily. Rooms with uncovered windows, bulletin boards with thematic pictures, and seasonal decorations can enhance time awareness. Person orientation can also be emphasized with environmental props. Color, shape, or object codes for each patient's clothing labels, furniture, and bedding can assist a patient in identifying possessions. Personalized symbols, such as a horse for a retired jockey, can serve as room or bed designations. Labelled family photographs, individual appointment calendars, and displays featuring a Patient-of-the-Month or Meet-a-Staff-Member are ways of highlighting individuality. A staff's creativity can add to this list of means by which the realities of time, person, place, and routines are advertised.

Two precautions should be taken when environmental props are used. The first is to establish responsibility for making certain the information is updated and accurate. Confused or disoriented patients may not recognize errors and yet have learned to depend on props for facts. The second precaution is against overzealous use of these props. Effectiveness is achieved when they are functional, simple, visually pleasant, and accessible. It is soon destroyed if the overall impact on the surroundings is a cluttered, chaotic, and clashing display.

Classroom RO. Structured lessons conducted by a trained leader are another facet of a Reality Orientation program. Emphasis continues to be placed on reinforcing the concepts of time, person, and place. Small, broadly homogeneous groups of four to six patients are assigned to either a basic or an advanced level class. Placement is a judgmental decision based on both objective and subjective evaluations of a patient's orientation, memory, and socialization skills and considerations of prognostic factors, physical limitations, and educational background. Originally, basic classes were scheduled daily for half an hour with advanced classes meeting for an hour (Folsom 1968). The length and frequency of classes may vary slightly but each patient should routinely attend them at least five days a week for the same thirty minutes each day (Drummond, Kirchhoff, and Scarbrough 1979).

Basic level classes are geared to patients whose orientation skills are minimal. Necessarily, the leader shoulders the primary responsibility for structuring exchanges between class members. Statements and questions are short, direct, and narrowly limit the choice of responses. Frequently, the correct answer is contained in the comment directed to a patient. Since response time may be quite slow, the leader must allow sufficient time for answers before proceeding. Feedback about responses is immediate and encouraging. Topical focus is kept to the immediate present, is concrete, and is restricted to one area of orientation at a time. Activities may include having the patient practice his or her name, repeating the leader's name, telling time by associating it with class times, reviewing each item on an RO board, and identifying familiar events or objects. Some biographical details from a patient's past are introduced when basic information is easily handled.

The advanced level classes contain elements of the basic skills but expand their use. The leader shares some responsibility for structuring exchanges by incorporating topics originating with class members. Comments directed to patients are more general and open thus permitting a wider choice of responses. Prompts are used minimally and less time is allowed before patients are expected to respond. Feedback to class members is delayed but remains encouraging. The focus of exchanges broadens to include past events, future expectations, more abstract associations, and a wholistic consideration of orienting information. Advanced groups learn the names of other class and staff members, practice clock-setting and telling time, associate times with various routines, complete personal appointment calendars, read maps, discuss seasonal activities, and make simple calculations.

As with other aspects of RO, Classroom RO has limitations. Leaders should be aware that conducting classes can be boring, repetitive work due to the practices of keeping materials and topics within the grasp of patients and consistently reiterating time-person-place information. Proponents of RO view these practices as necessary but recognize their drawbacks to leaders. Further, patient behaviors can create problems for a leader yet need resolution if the rest of the group is to function well. Periodic rotation of classroom assignments, supportive and enthusiastic supervision, and adequate training are seen as solutions to these disadvantages. Another limitation is experienced if complementary emphasis on orientation and application of RO guidelines away from the classroom is lacking. Group activities may be considered, at best, diversional and purposeless by both classroom leaders and participants. Gubrium and Ksander (1975) described such a situation as observed in two nursing homes. Their critique should ring a cautionary note to those who would implement a RO program in a mechanistic fashion with neither an empathetic appreciation for each patient's individuality, worth, dignity, and needs nor a solid foundation of staff support and cooperation. Finally, expectations for the benefits classroom work may hold have to be realistic. Leaders must be aware of the general prognosis and goals established for patients, complications for which compensations are feasible, how the class fits in with other rehabilitative efforts, and the options available for patients once they master advanced level material. Without a realistic context for themselves, leaders may become disheartened and begin to doubt their effectiveness or their worth in the care of confused or disoriented individuals.

Behavioral management. Another feature of RO is the sensitization of staff members to the effects their attitudes have on patients' behavior generally and the means by which consistent and conscious use of certain expressed attitudes can alter patients' problematic behavior. The assumption is made that attitudes are contagious. For example, should one person relate to another in a constantly bored and superficial manner, it is expected that the reactions will eventually reflect this treatment, perhaps taking the form of undesired withdrawal and apathy. According to Drummond et al. (1978), "active friendliness is used in approaching the confused person. This is a supportive, ego-building attitude that helps the person to feel that he is worth something. . . " The responsibility for altering attitudes and their behavioral correlates is placed on each staff member; however, patients must also learn to assume control of their behavior. It is proposed that the latter is assisted by the type of responses staff members consistently give to undesirable behavior.

A distinction is made between sudden and unexpected shifts in a patient's behavior and a general pattern a patient has developed over time. For the former, the primary concern is safety for the patient and people around him or her if the shift is toward violence. Otherwise, supportive acknowledgement of the underlying emotions accompanied by an attitude that conveys responsibility for behavior to the patient is considered an appropriate reaction. By applying the recommendations for twenty-four hour RO, most sudden changes to an undesirable behavior can be managed satisfactorily.

Maladaptive patterns of behavior are approached by prescribing certain attitudes for the entire staff to use whenever the undesirable behavior occurs. Five patterns are so predominant that they have been singled out and general management guidelines have been suggested (AHA 1973). Withdrawn patients are consistently treated in an outgoing, friendly manner with initiative for conversations or activity assumed by the staff members. Patients who display a pattern of distrustfulness are purposefully given the initiative to interact with others. Members of the staff express friendliness when approached by this type of patient but are noncommittal and avoid pushing the patient into decisions. Quarrelsome individuals receive a firm, matter-of-fact attitude. Since it requires two people to quarrel, the staff avoids being drawn into arguments. Persons who have developed a depressed behavioral pattern are related to kindly but firmly. Conscious efforts are made to help the depressed patients alter their preoccupation with themselves by refocusing their attention to meaningful activities involving others. Finally, the staff in an RO program handles complaining, manipulative patients by using a matter-of-fact attitude and being resistent to the patients' inappropriate attempts to manipulate them.

Family RO. The final and equally important aspect of RO is the involvement of family and/or close friends in the treatment program. An early emphasis is placed on assisting them to overcome the feelings of guilt, hopelessness, pity, and sorrow that frequently arise when a loved one is in need of long-term care. An educational phase promotes an understanding of the aging process, common faulty assumptions about aging, the nature of confusion and disorientation, and the philosophies of rehabilitation. The training segment teaches the seven fundamental guidelines for reorienting confused and disoriented individuals and provides support as they are put into practice. Private meetings with families cover the particulars of diagnosis, prognosis, treatment plans, the rationale behind decisions, and the types of activities the family can promote. These meetings are ideal for obtaining detailed background information on a patient's preferences, hobbies, special memories, former habits and preferred routines which the staff, in turn, can attempt to honor and incorporate into the patient's life at their facility. Frequent visits with their loved ones are encouraged and, when feasible, short excursions from the facility are planned. When a patient is discharged, the staff continues in the role of a resource on which the family can depend for guidance. The aims of this family involvement are to ease the transition into a non-home setting, to provide a sound base for continuing family ties, and to enlist the family as supportive members of the treatment team.

Summary

Reality Orientation is not a comprehensive answer to all issues of geriatric care. It is a technique proposed specifically for individuals described as confused and/or disoriented. As with any approach, its merits and limitations must be considered in the light of a particular person's needs and the resources available within a particular setting for implementing an RO program. To be effective, stimulation must be adequate and staff functions must be both coordinated and cooperative. Its stability as a technique is based on a fidelity to seven guidelines which stress certain environmental, social, contextual, behavioral, and attitudinal tenets. Its versatility is the result of the varied patient populations and settings to which it can be adapted, the purposes it serves, and the combinations that can be effected when choices among the five features of a complete RO program must be made.

PRACTICAL CONSIDERATIONS FOR ESTABLISHING AN RO PROGRAM

The American Hospital Association (1973) has produced a thorough, detailed resource for those people seeking to establish RO in their facility. It includes several readings of general and specific relevance to RO, assessment forms, a plan for implementing a program, and a complete training module for introducing RO to a staff. Other obtainable resources (Drummond et al., 1978; Hefferin and Hunter 1977; Lee 1976 a and b; Stephens 1969) are less detailed but contain useful descriptions and suggestions. Both Cornbleth and Cornbleth (1977) and Drummond et al. (1979) have provided detailed guides for Classroom RO. The most up-to-date information and training opportunities are available through the Reality Orientation Training Program, Veterans Administration Hospital, Tuscaloosa, Alabama 35401, which also publishes a newsletter to keep practioners informed on recent publications, material resources, educational opportunities, and noteworthy ideas. These avenues of preparation provide a solid foundation on which to plan an RO program to complement any setting offering services to confused or disoriented patients.

Securing administrative approval and support is generally the first step taken toward introducing RO as an additional approach to patient care. When an administration is skeptical, it is helpful to (a) describe the intent, scope, and versatility of RO, (b) share the research findings that are available, (c) estimate the number of patients for whom RO would be appropriate, (d) identify current procedures that could be readily included or easily adapted to an RO approach, and (e) detail likely changes or additions to current procedures. Requests for administrative sanction are further enhanced by presenting a tentative outline of each implementation stage which summarizes the rationale and goals for each step and gives an anticipated timetable, the expected staff commitments, and cost estimates. The most substantial investment when beginning an RO program is in staff time. Cash outlays occur primarily for meeting the educational needs of those who will be training the facility's staff, procuring instructional materials for classes, obtaining necessary forms, and making some environmental improvements. Such options as conducting case studies or a pilot project may be more appealing to some administrations and can be pursued. These approaches provide important data and, in the case of a pilot project, also reveal potential problem areas. Such information can prove useful when a broader program is attempted. Finally, it is essential to the smooth operation of RO to have one person assigned the responsibility for coordinating the details of implementation and the personnel to be involved. This individual will require authority to make and act on decisions affecting the program and must have administrative support and recognition.

Once administrative approval is secured and a coordinator is appointed, specific policies and procedures are developed. Several determinations may have been made during discussions with the administration or as outgrowths of either a pilot project or case studies. Many options are available so decisions can be compatible with and enhance established procedures. Because staff selection and training are pivotal to any program, these are early concerns for the coordinator. The beliefs and funds of information each staff member will represent are important determinants through which the tenets of RO will be interpreted and practiced. Where negativism, large differences in background or experience, and substantial disagreements between disciplines are apparent, RO training would be wisely deferred until a preliminary emphasis can be given to: (a) pertinent facts about the aging process, (b) factors influencing mental faculties, (c) the impact of attitudes on human behaivor, (d) general terminology, and (e) multidisciplinary team philosophies and practices. Both Palmore (1977) and the AHA (1973) offer material designed to explore attitudinal and factual variations within a staff which instructiors can use to promote discussions. A successfully instituted RO program will be partially dependent on attaining some shared points of reference so that a staff can function as a multidisciplinary team characterized by mutual respect for one another's perspectives and contributions.

A cohesive treatment team can become a valuable resource for the individual responsible for devising RO procedures. Members can reviw materials and share ideas for making the procedures compatible with the realistic capacity of the team. Since these are the individuals who will be analyzing, appraising, diagnosing, and treating the patients, their considered opinions, as reflected in the coordinator's decisions, will form the basis of support for advancing the program. The major issues to brainstorm are: (a) the specific responsibilities of each member, (b) the means by which appropriate patients will be identified and referred to the program, (c) the criteria, if any, by which patients will be enrolled, (d) the appraisal tools to be used, (e) the frequency of reevaluations, (f) the standards for advancing or discharging patients, (g) the frequency and format of team conferences, (h) the communication channels for informing the staff about current patient status, (i) the logistics for transporting patients and assigning leaders to Classroom RO, (j) the number, types, and locations of environmental props, and (k) the kinds of activities for promoting family involvement. Two of these concerns, patient criteria and appraisal, are singled out for additional comments.

At our facility, we have established an RO program for which referral and intake criteria have been specified. They were developed eclectically from the above-mentioned sources, research findings, and our experiences with a one-year pilot project. One purpose of these criteria is to identify the patients who are most likely to benefit from RO techniques and who will provide added motivation to our staff through their improvement. Our second purpose is to select patients with whom a solid foundation of skills and procedures can be built before we introduce more challenging, difficult patients to our program. The referral criteria and rationales are:

1. The onset of confusion or disorientation was sudden but may have occurred at any time relative to the present. Patients with degenerative diseases are the group eliminated by this criterion. Although our preference is for early identification and referral, by not specifying a minimum time since onset, those patients who may have deteriorated for other than medical reasons remain eligible for referral.

2. Etiology is nonpsychiatric, e.g., is not catatonic schizophrenia. Since our facility has a psychiatric ward with specialized staff, this criterion is intended to eliminate patients most appropriately cared for by their team. Inservice training has been provided on RO principles and techniques so they may be applied when valid.

3. Medically treatable causes have been eliminated or controlled. This attempts to assure that symptoms of confusion or disorientation have become chronic and will require rehabilitation efforts if improvement is to be made.

4. The patient is medically stable. Since frequent fluxuations in a patient's health status can seriously disrupt a plan of care and make a routine difficult to maintain, this criterion eliminates patients who could not dependably participate in rehabilitative activities.

5. Sensory impairments (hearing and vision) are corrected and/or are of moderate to mild severity. This prerequisite is intended to rule out deafness or blindness. As we broaden our program, it is anticipated that compensatory techniques will be devised so that such patients will be accepted into the program.

6. The patient's speech is sufficiently intelligible to permit a listener to recognize most words used in short sentences. Two purposes are served by this requirement: to screen out patients who have significant communication disorders complicating or camouflaging confusion and disorientation and to increase the likelihood of a patient being testable.

7. Interpersonal behavior is appropriate enough to permit the patient to function in a small group. This last referral criterion eliminates patients whose behavioral patterns, e.g. violence, constitute a major barrier to intervention for the patient and an unfair disruption to other patients' activities.

When referral criteria are met or when doubt exists, a consultation giving the pertinent, broad etiological category, the diagnosis, and the approximate date of onset is sent to the RO coordinator. The medical record is reviewed and the patient is screened for severity using Pfeiffer's Short Portable Mental Status Questionnaire, the spatial relations subtest from the Reitan-Indiana Aphasia Screening Test, and a self-evaluation questionnaire developed by our team. If a patient's scores fall within the range of two to eight errors on the first two screening measures, i.e. moderately severe confusion and/or disorientation is likely, the patient is recommended for the RO program. If either referral or intake criteria are failed, it is noted on the consultation request and other recommendations are offered. Reconsultation is urged if disqualifying factors are eliminated.

Appraisal can become a burden if several considerations are overlooked. The staff's attitude will be important and will generally be supportive when the purpose is clear, the resulting information is meaningfully utilized, and new procedures with any ensuing forms are complementary to existing protocols rather than a duplication of efforts. Unless practicality is a characteristic, a program will risk having good appraisal procedures that are seldom honored once they are incorporated into other duties the staff members will have. For example, three sets each averaging a ten-minute administration time may be selected and two aides assigned the responsibility for administering them. This reasonable decision could become cumbersome if reassessment is scheduled weekly for twenty-five patients since an estimated total of twelve & a half hours, or over 15% of each aide's forty-hour duty tour, would be devoted to data collection alone. Assessment tools must also meet the scope of RO. Since it is designed to impact confusion, disorientation, and dependency in a context of keen appreciation for the individual, these constitute the most pertinent areas for appraisal. Typically, orientation is assessed by a verbal questionnaire (AHA 1973; Cornbleth and Cornbleth 1977). Erickson et al. (1978) suggested written questionnaires or multiple choice tests for capable patients to complete. Since patients can give certain answers on tests yet behave differently than their answers would imply, direct observation of patients during daily activities supplements formal testing. Direct observations are usually recorded on a functional rating scale. Several are included in the research on RO and the AHA (1973) material contains a scale developed for the Reality Orientation program in Tuscaloosa, Alabama. Cornbleth (1978) devised the Geriatric Resident Goals Scale, a checklist of eighty-five specific behavioral goals arranged under six categorical headings, which may be used to determine a patient's current status, to develop treatment goals, and to evaluate a plan's effectiveness by periodically reassessing a patient's abilities. Detailed social histories provide essential personalizing information. Erickson et al. (1978) suggested assessing avocational interests for individualizing recreational activities. Of course, several other aspects of mental, emotional, physical, and sensory abilities are relevant, for instance memory capacity, and data about them are highly desirable. This desire for a variety of data may require a compromise, however, where time and personnel constraints exist. Our program has restricted its assessment to a verbal orientation questionnaire, the Geriatric Resident Goals Scale, and a detailed medical/social history. Any special concerns arising out of an analysis of this data are handled through consultation requests sent to appropriate services within the hospital.

Once most policies and procedures have been determined, the next phase of implementation is training. Prepared instructional materials for introducing RO to a staff can be well utilized if previewed and adapted to fit a particular setting's decisions. Training is offered to all staff members who will be expected to carry out the various aspects of RO. Even those people involved with the initial decision-making can benefit from instruction that conveys the flow of the whole program. In the event that training is provided to individuals who do not view themselves in direct patient care roles, some stress is appropriately placed on their special contributions and opportunities for giving such care. People who escort patients to appointments are one such group. They can provide time and place orientation, in particular, and can serve as liaisons between patients' living areas and clinics. Instruction for them could highlight twenty-four hour RO techniques and the tenet of consistency. Staff members who either volunteer or are assigned for classroom duties are another group for whom instructors can adapt training to correspond with anticipated functions. Our experience made us realize that meaningful preparation for RO is most likely when participants understand the overall context into which their duties fit and acquire specific information about how their duties will change. Tailoring the training to fit the audience does require advanced planning and some preparation of original materials but is well-rewarded when a consensus of support, a willingness to accommodate, and a knowledge of program expectations are gained.

For a new RO program, the next step of actually beginning it with patients will entail coordination so that patient participants are conveniently grouped, essential environmental props are in place, the classroom is equipped, personnel schedules are established, and necessary forms are completed. This is a time when more frequent team meetings and, perhaps, special sessions with homogeneous staff, i.e. all nursing assistants, may be held so that concerns, problems, and ideas can be readily shared. Supervisory encouragement and recognition of initiative help motivate and interest staff until their efforts are reflected in the patients themselves. As the various procedures and techniques become part of accepted routine, meetings may decrease in frequency without a breakdown in côordination. One advantage of careful appraisal and record keeping can be demonstrated as soon as the first reassessment period is completed. By sharing the results of the staff's efforts in identifying and enrolling patients in the program, reporting on class attendance, discussing comparative data collected, and detailing any other information routinely obtained, the RO coordinator can keep staff members informed about the value of their varied contributions. Continued periodic feedback can further underscore staff accomplishments in their patient care activities.

While family members and close friends continue their usual visits, the phase of comprehensive family education should be delayed long enough for the facility's staff to become accustomed to any changes in their duties and their ways of interacting with patients. Printed information describing the program, giving suggestions, and listing some helpful techniques for the family to follow is usefully introduced as soon as RO is recommended for a patient. Questions can be answered during private sessions when social history is taken and again after a treatment plan has been devised. Once the program is operational, more extensive and formal sessions with families may be introduced. Should family members and friends be unavailable, too distant, or no longer living, other alternatives for companionship visits could be explored and persons thus identified would receive training. Some suggestions that emerged from our pilot project were to have a family information center on a bulletin board, a single contact person assigned to each shift to answer family concerns, and self-study materials to supplement formal sessions. Families soon become another source of ideas when their contributions are supported and appreciated. In our opinion, they are the very real symbols for sustaining hope and aspiration in patients since it is through their continuing concern and assistance that a patient's genuine significance to others is demonstrated.

SUMMARY

An expanded understanding of normal aging processes and the acceptance of a positive attitude toward problems experienced by elderly individuals have prompted concern for improving services rendered to them. For those older citizens who experience confusion and/or disorientation associated with disease, psychological difficulties, sensory deprivation, and environmental incompatibility, the outlook is no longer without hope or without help. Once etiological and diagnostic determinations are made, principles and techniques collectively referred to as Reality Orientation can be applied to assist these people in reorienting themselves. Reality Orientation is premised on the assumptions that direct, active, and positive psychotherapeutic intervention stressing stimulation, repetition, structure and consistency will alleviate and reverse the deterioration often associated with chronic confusion and disorientation. Research gives general support to these beliefs but the relationships between orientation and self-sufficiency in daily activities are not clearly established. Reality Orientation programs are necessarily multidisciplinary and have versatility which give the approach broad appeal. It is based on seven fundamental principles which are employed while communicating with patients, developing and using environmental props, conducting orientation classes, managing behavioral problems, and assisting family members to care for their loved ones. Assuring a successfully founded program is dependent on securing administrative approval, having an appointed coordinator, attaining shared points of reference between multidisciplinary staff members, establishing a broad base of support, developing viable policies and procedures, providing adequate, relevant training, and monitoring program activities. The ultimate worth of a Reality Orientation program in any setting will have to be judged by the patients, families, and staff who are working together to facilitate a better reality for their lives.

References

American Hospital Association. *This way to reality: guide for developing a reality orientation program.* Washington, D.C.: National Audiovisual Center (GSA), 1973. (Audiotapes, Slides, Notebook)

Barnes, J. A. Effects of reality orientation classroom on memory loss, confusion and disorientation in geriatric patients. *The Gerontologist,* 1974, *14:* 138-142.

Brook, P., Degun, G., & Mather, M. Reality orientation, a therapy for psychogeriatric patients: a controlled study. *British Journal of Psychiatry,* 1975, *127:* 42-45.

Burnside, I. M. Reality testing: an important concept. *American Rehabilitation Nursing Journal,* 1977, *2* (3): 3-4, 6-7, 9.

Cape, R. D. *Aging: its complex management.* New York: Harper & Row Publishers, Inc., 1978.

Citrin, R. S. & Dixon, D. N. Reality orientation: a milieu therapy used in an institution for the aged. *The Gerontologist,* 1977, *17:* 39-43.

Cornbleth, T. Evaluation of goal attainment in geriatric settings. *Journal of the American Geriatrics Society*, 1978, *26:* 404-407.

Cornbleth, T. & Cornbleth, C. Reality orientation for the elderly. JSAS *Catalogue of Selected Documents in Psychology*, 1977, 7, 80. (Ms. No. 1539.)

Cornbleth, T. & Cornbleth, C. Evaluation of the effectiveness of reality orientation classes in a nursing home unit. *Journal of the American Geriatrics Society*, 1979, *27:* 522-524.

Drummond, L., Kirchhoff, L., & Scarbrough, D. A practical guide to reality orientation: a treatment approach for confusion and disorientation. *The Gerontologist*, 1978, *18:* 568-573.

Drummond, L., Kirchhoff, L., & Scarbrough, D. R. *Leading reality orientation classes: basic and advanced.* Tuscaloosa, Alabama: VA Medical Center Manual Arts Therapy, 1979.

Erickson, R., English, S., Halar, E., & Hibbert, J. Employing reality orientation in a short term treatment setting. *American Rehabilitation Nursing Journal*, 1978, *3* (6): 18-21.

Folsom, J. C. Reality orientation for the elderly mental patient. *Journal of Geriatric Psychiatry*, 1968, *1:* 291-307.

Greene, J. C., Nicol, R., & Jamieson, H. Reality orientation with psychogeriatric patients. *Behavior Research and Therapy*, 1979, *17:* 615-618.

Gubrium, J. F. & Ksander, M. On multiple realities and reality orientation. *The Gerontologist*, 1975, *15:* 142-145.

Hackley, J. A. Reality orientation brings patients back from confusion and apathy. *Modern Nursing Home,* September 1973: 48-49.

Harris, C. S. & Ivory, P. B. C. B. An outcome evaluation of reality orientation therapy with geriatric patients in a state mental hospital. *The Gerontologist*, 1976, *16:* 496-503.

Hefferin, E. A. & Hunter, R. E. How we turned the idea into a program: reality orientation. *Nursing*, May 1977: 89-91, 93-94.

Hogstel, M. O. Use of reality orientation with aging confused patients. *Nursing Research*, 1979, *28:* 161-165.

Holden, U. P. & Sinebruchow, A. Reality orientation therapy: a study investigating the value of this therapy in the rehabilitation of elderly people. *Age and Aging*, 1978, *7:* 83-90.

Isler, C. Who says senile geriatric patients are untreatable? *RN,* June 1975: 39-50.

Jahraus, A. M. Who is confused? *Nursing Homes,* August-September 1974: 6-9.

Katz, M. M. Behavior change in the chronicity pattern of dementia in the institutional geriatric resident. *Journal of the American Geriatrics Society*, 1976, *24:* 522-528.

Lee, R. E. Reality orientation: restoring the senile to life (part 1). *Journal of Practical Nursing*, 1976a, *26,* (1): 28-29, 35, 37.

Lee, R. E. Reality orientation: restoring the senile to life (part 2). *Journal of Practical Nursing*, 1976b, *26* (2): 30-31.

Letcher, P. B., Peterson, L. P., & Scarbrough, D. Reality orientation: a historical study of patient progress. *Hospital & Community Psychiatry*, 1974, *25:* 801-803.

MacDonald, M. L. & Settin, J. M. Reality orientation versus sheltered workshops as treatment for the institutionalized aging. *Journal of Gerontology*, 1978, *33:* 416-421.

Palmore, E. Facts on aging: a short quiz. *The Gerontologist,* 1977, *17:* 315-320.

Phillips, D. F. Reality orientation: a new therapeutic mode. *Hospitals,* July 1973: 46-49, 101.

Scarbrough, D. Reality orientation: a new approach to an old problem. *Nursing,* November 1974: 12-13.

Stephens, L. P., ed. Reality orientation: a technique to rehabilitate elderly and brain damaged patients with a moderate to severe degree of disorientation. Washington, D.C.: American Psychiatric Association, 1969.

Taulbee, L. R. Reorientation means independence and dignity. *Modern Nursing Home,* September 1973: 50-51.

Voelkel, D. A study of reality orientation and resocialization groups with confused elderly. *Journal of Gerontological Nursing,* 1978, *4* (3): 13-18.

Wertz, R. T. Neuropathologies in speech and language: an introduction to patient management. In D. F. Johns (ed.), *Clinical Management of Neurogenic Communicative Disorders.* Boston: Little, Brown & Co., 1978.

Woods, R. T. Reality Orientation and staff attention: a controlled study. *British Journal of Psychiatry,* 1979, 134: 502-507.

Woods, R. T. & Britton, P. G. Psychological approaches to the treatment of the elderly. *Age and Aging,* 1977, *6:* 104-112.

6

The Role of Bibliotherapy and Reading for the Aging

George M. Usova

Bibliotherapy, as a mental health intervention approach, is a significant and growing mode of therapy for assisting the aging. Present day educators commonly use bibliotherapy with children and youth in classroom settings. In this regard, bibliotherapy is used in both a developmental and remedial sense. Teachers have used and continue to use bibliotherapy in a developmental sense by guiding and directing students toward ready literature which has positive values toward social-emotional development; teacher-pupil discussion toward the integration of conceptual ideas and values within the individual enhances personal development. In its remedial sense, teachers employ the technique to reduce social-emotional problems by directing youth to those ready materials which may provide for an identification, an empathy, or a catharsis to the individual problem, and thereby create the understanding for a solution.

In its basic intent, the use of bibliotherapy for the aging is no different than that used for youth. There are, to be certain, other differences which lie primarily in the unique needs and setting of the aging. The aging, as a significantly growing segment of the population, will bring about a different set of problems than those encountered by youth. The role of bibliotherapy as an approach to the development of improved mental health or to the improvement of poor mental health will need to interface with concerns of physical disabilities, hospital or nursing home settings, delivery of services, qualified staff to provide this approach, and a host of social-economic-political issues.

This chapter was written by George M. Usova in his private capacity. No official support or endorsement by the U.S. Department of Education is intended or should be inferred.

While bibliotherapy is not a new concept, its application to the aging is; the possibilities of its success and impact are exciting. The mental health practitioner needs to know more about the approach and its inter-relationship to the field of reading and the aging. This chapter will focus on providing this information by addressing the following areas: defining bibliotherapy and discussing its application; reviewing research findings in the field of reading as it relates to the aged; examining approaches in im-plementing bibliotherapy in various group settings; and exploring future needs and trends of bibliotherapy for the aging.

BIBLIOTHERAPY DEFINED

Bibliotherapy has been described by Monroe (1971) as part of a continuum of library services. Reference, reading guidance and bibliotherapy are closely related in function. All three serve informational, instructional and/or guidance needs. Reference services are objective, informational and of short duration, while reading guidance is subjective and more broadly educational. Bibliotherapy is a long-term approach to library services for therapeutic purposes. This concept of bibliotherapy as an outgrowth of reader's services is accepted also by Hannigan (1962): "This skill [bibliotherapy] is a refined application of his normal librarian's function as readers' advisor." Tews (1962), in an expanded definition defines bibliotherapy as

> a program of selected activity involving reading materials, planned, conducted, and controlled as treatment under the guidance of the physician for emotional and other problems. It must be administered by a skilled, professionally trained librarian with prescribed purpose and goals. The important and dynamic factors are the relationships which are established, the patient's reactions and responses, and the reporting back to the physician for interpretation, evaluation, and direction in follow-up.

In its current state, bibliotherapy is usually practiced with a group. It can therefore be considered as an outgrowth of the field of group psychology, which made large strides during 1920-40. The term "group therapy" was coined in 1931. Psychodrama was introduced in 1925 and dance therapy in 1942. By the 1950s, with the advent of art and music therapies, the idea of creative, adjunctive, group therapy was well ac-cepted. Adult education, which flourished in the 1930s and 1940s, also claims to be a precursor to bibliotherapy. The book-based discussion groups exemplified by the Great Books program of 1945 paralleled the more therapy-oriented service called bibliotherapy. The interdisciplinary background of bibliotherapy can be clearly illustrated by an analysis of its recent literature. Of the 131 articles published from 1970 to 1975, 35%

appeared in library journals and 65% in periodicals of other fields such as psychology, education, nursing and occupational therapy.

The term *bibliotherapy* is derived from the Greek *biblion* (book) and *therapeia* (healing). Samuel McChord Crothers coined the word in a 1916 Atlantic Monthly article, and there has been confusion about it ever since. In 1961, *Webster's Third New International Dictionary* published the definition which was officially accepted in 1966 by ALA: "the use of selected reading materials as therapeutic adjuvants in medicine and in psychiatry; also: guidance in the solution of personal problems through directed reading." Rubin (1979) prefers to define bibliotherapy as: "a program of activity based on the interactive processes of media and the people who experience it. Print or non-print material, either imaginative or informational, is experienced and discussed with the aid of a facilitator." This concept includes the application of bibliotherapy in institutional or community settings, via print as well as other media, using didactic or imaginative literature in programs under the direction of one or more professionals. Its goal is either insight into normal development or changes in disturbed behavior. Since the definition—and the field—is so broad, a three-pronged approach to bibliotherapy through classification according to participants, goals, settings and leaders has been adopted.

The three types of bibliotherapy are institutional, clinical and developmental. Institutional bibliotherapy is the direct descendant of bibliotherapy as practiced in the 1930s by psychiatrists (notably William Menninger). It refers to the reading of literature (usually didactic) by institutionalized patients who then discuss it with the doctor. The phrase "prescription of books for specific ills" applies to this approach. The goal is primarily informational, although some insight materials may be offered; the setting is an institution; and the facilitator is a physician or a medical team which may include a librarian. This type of bibliotherapy is not popular today, although some doctors still use media with individual patients in their private practice.

Clinical bibliotherapy refers to the use of imaginative literature with groups of clients with emotional or behavioral problems. The goals range from insight to change in behavior; the setting is either an institution or the community; and the facilitator is either a librarian or a doctor, usually in consultation with the other. Exemplary clinical bibliotherapy programs are ongoing at St. Elizabeths Hospital in Washington, D.C., and at the Santa Clara County Free Library in San Jose, California.

Developmental bibliotherapy refers to the use of both imaginative and didactic materials with groups of "normal" individuals. The goal is to promote normal development and self-actualization or to maintain mental health. This type of bibliotherapy is often provided in schools, libraries and other community settings. The program discussion is designed and led by a librarian, teacher or other member of the "helping professions," such as a social worker or psychologist. Developmental bibliotherapy is the approach most often used by public librarians and the one that can most readily be used in response to three societal trends that is, it can be utilized as part of consciousness-raising, or sensitivity training programs for professionals, or offered as a public program to satisfy the demand for self-actualization activities.

Franklin Berry (1978) proceeds to define and further delineate the elements of bibliotherapy. He states that contemporary bibliotherapy is not a well-articulated or coherent field. It is instead a multifarious collection of techniques and practices in which literature is used in some fashion to structure or organize interpersonal interactions. These techniques and practices are all based on the sharing of literature; the bibliotherapist and her participants directly experience some form of literature and they discuss its significance to their lives. In these discussions they initially share their ideas, their feelings and their perspectives aroused by the literature they have mutually experienced; then, the act of sharing itself allows each person to receive *feedback* from others concerning his/her own unique perception of the experienced literature. The feedback received may be of the direct kind—one person making specific comments to another about the former's ideas/feelings/perspectives which were ostensibly aroused by the mutually experienced literature; or it may be of the indirect kind—one person relates his/her ideas/feelings/perspectives about the shared literature and another listens to this report and compares his/her own perceptions to the former's.

Whether of the direct or indirect kind, the feedback received during the bibliotherapy process seems to be extremely important. A participant initially interprets a literary selection in light of his/her own past history, then, as a result of others' sharing of their perspectives, the literature-as-interpreted is reexperienced and may then come to evoke additional meanings and associated feelings. Of course, the direct kind of feedback may also convey others' perceptions of a given participant ("dishonest," "warm," "intolerant," "friendly"), as well as their perceptions of his/her shared ideas/feelings/perspectives. These other points of view can also be presented explicitly—"You are not being honest about how you feel about that poem."—or implicitly—"Are you sure that that's how you feel about that poem?"

Given the previous discussion, the following definition is offered for contemporary bibliotherapy:

> Bibliotherapy refers to a family of techniques in which *literature* is used in some way to structure or organize interactions between a facilitator (or co-facilitators) and a *participant* (or a group of participants), where the term literature is to be interpreted in the broadest

sense possible, where the goal of the process is to benefit the participants in some fashion and where the facilitator, serving as a change-agent, actively attempts to realize his/her goals (and/or the participants' goals).

Given this working definition of bibliotherapy, it becomes apparent that the principal ingredients of bibliotherapy consist of (a) the literature which shapes, determines, or colors the nature of the interpersonal interactions, either as initially experienced or as reexperienced following feedback from others' perceptions of the same literature; (b) the bibliotherapist/facilitator (or facilitators); and (c) the bibliotherapy-participant (or participants).

It should be noted also that the differentiation of facilitator versus participant roles implies a difference in power/authority/responsibility between the persons playing these different roles and also that the persons involved have different sets of expectations for each by virtue of their respective roles. That is to say, our working definition implies that: the facilitator leads the interaction and/or determines the form that the interaction takes; and that the participant follows the lead of the facilitator and is aware of the fact that the facilitator is to some extent controlling the form of the interaction.

This definition of bibliotherapy also makes explicit the fact that the facilitator has specific goals which s/he wants to accomplish as a consequence of the bibliotherapeutic experience. The implication here, of course, is that the facilitator is actively working to facilitate some change in the participants; further, s/he is (by definition) aware that the power of literature is being harnessed to effect the desired change in the particpants (coupled, of course, with the power of feedback from a significant other, e.g., the facilitator or another particpant, for producing reinterpretations of the previously experienced literature and concomitantly changes in participants' perspectives.).

While the definition offered for contemporary bibliotherapy is not wholly satisfactory, it does possess a number of useful features. One particularly useful feature of the definition is that it is general enough to subsume bibliotherapy practices based on the sharing of preexisting literature as well as those based on the sharing of participant-created literature. One has only to consider the great diversity of "preexisting literature," from written poetry, short stories, plays, novels, and so on, to oral literary traditions like fables, folk tales, legends, myths, parables, and so on, to begin to appreciate the extremely wide scope of the proffered definition. Contemporary bibliotherapy sessions are frequently based on the sharing of an equally diverse assortment of "participant-created literature" (from written poems, short stories, reminiscenses, personal journals, life reviews to oral versions of these same literary forms, and so on), and an even clearer picture emerges of the purview of the definition of bibliotherapy under consideration here. Thus, bibliotherapy has both experience-preexisting-literature-and-discuss-it characteristics *and* create-literature-and-discuss-it characteristics, and both approaches are based on diverse literary forms.

These aspects of contemporary bibliotherapy are elaborated in Table 1 in conjunction with two other important dimensions of any bibliotherapy experience: (a) the nature of the literature experienced (*written literature versus oral literature* for the preexisting literature dimension; or *literature created-in-writing* versus *literature created-orally* for the created literature dimension); and (b) the nature of the participant's literature experience (*experienced/created in session,* or *experienced/created outside session*

The analysis offered in Table 1 constitutes an integration of bibliotherapy based on preexisting literature (referred to there as emphasizing the participant's receptive language response system) and bibliotherapy based on participant-created literature (referred to there as emphasizing the participant's expressive language response system) with the dimension of the nature of the literature experience cited above. The systematization proposed in Table 1 subsumes the subdivision of bibliotherapy referred to as the "field of poetry therapy", for the most part within cell A: Reading-discussion poetry therapy. (See Poetry Therapy Readings at the end of the chapter for a detailed bibliography of poetry therapy).

Given the analysis to follow in which the nature of the participant's literature experience is explored, one finds that all of the following qualify as bibliotherapy based upon preexisiting literature according to the extremely broad conceptual approach to the field taken here:

1. Reading-discussion group in which the participant's reading experience takes place during the group meeting in which the material is discussed with the facilitator and other participants.

2. Oral-discussion group in which the participant's listening to oral literature or written literature presented orally takes place during the group meeting in which the material is discussed with the facilitator and other participants.

3. Reading-discussion group in which the participant's reading experience is completed prior to the group meeting and is followed up by subsequent discussion of what was read with the facilitator and the other participants.

4. Oral-discussion group in which the participant's listening to oral literature or written literature presented orally (say, as a tape recording) is completed prior to the group meeting and is followed up by subsequent discussion of what was heard with the facilitator and other participants.

The field of "reading" is obviously an integral part of the biblio-

Table 1.   Nature of the Participant's Literature Experience[a]

Receptive Language Experience

	Experienced In Session	Experienced Outside Session
Written Literature	A[b]	A
Oral Literature	A	A

(left axis label: Preexisting Literature)

Expressive Language Experience

	Created In Session	Created Outside Session
Created In Writing	A′	A′
Created Orally	A[b]′	A′

(left axis label: Created Literature)

[a] Note that this analysis assumes that the participant and the facilitator share the literature that they have mutually experienced in a face to face encounter.

[b] Note also that A and A′ represent literature experiences with a specific literary genre. A represents a literary piece existing in the world's literature, and A′ a comparable literary piece created by a participant as an integral part of the bibliotherapy experience.

therapy approach. Of primary importance, is an understanding of the reading interests, habits, and attitudes of the aged. The practitioner needs to consider the integration of reading with therapy in light of available research.

When one thinks of remaining mentally active during the aging process, one of the activities that comes to mind is reading. Research relative to the reading interests of older adults is scarce (Kingston 1979; De Santi 1976; Robinson and Maring 1976); this is not surprising. Perhaps this reflects an attitude of society relative to the young versus the old—the young are catered to and the old are either tolerated or ignored (De Santi 1976). In fact, Tuckman and Lorge (1952) found that by the age of ten, children have developed a negative view of aging. More recently, Ansello (1977) cited numerous studies with young children, older children and adolescents, and with older adults themselves in which the predominant view of aging seemed to be negative.

Nevertheless, with the increasing acceptance of adult education as a field of study and the emergence of the concept of lifelong learning, the educational spotlight is now focusing on the adult segment of society, including older adults. Furthermore, there has been a remarkable increase in the number of older persons, and this has been a major determinant in the increased interest in the aging population (De Santi 1976).

REVIEW OF THE STUDIES

Moshey (1972) studied fifty retired adults, ten males and forty females, in New Jersey. They were considered to be middle or upper middle-class former professionals. She found that their preference of reading material included biographies, travel books, and fiction. Furthermore, all of the males and 90% of the females read the newspaper.

In a survey of 5,000 noninstitutionalized adults, those over sixty read more books than did the group from forty to sixty years of age (Riley and Foner 1968). The amount of leisure time used for reading tends to increase as adults grow older; however, idleness consumes most of the time, especially in the lowest income group.

The fact that the lowest income group apparently does little reading is not surprising in light of the fact that this group is generally less educated as well. Also, those persons over sixty-five have less education than younger adults due in part to the era in which they were born (Eklund 1969). Of these adults 76% have completed eight years or less of formal education, and many fall into the nearly illiterate category. More than 20% have four years or less of schooling, an educational level that does little to aid them in coping with everyday life in this modern technological society; nor does it prepare them intellectually to do much reading.

The situation is probably worse than it appears in that these, some twenty million adults referred to above indicated the level of schooling completed. However, there is a vast difference in the level of school completed and one's educational "functional" level. One may have completed the tenth grade; but when tested for actual reading skills, one's reading level may only be the third grade. Thus, the lower the reading level, the more difficult it is to read the books and magazines available.

Romani (1973) found that the aged prefer reading material that deals with light romance and no sex, biographies, books in biographies, books in large print, westerns, and mysteries. They do not care for science fiction or books containing violence. In addition, they have less need for vocational or professional reading materials.

Wilson (1979) reports the results of "Readarama," a series of sessions held one-hour weekly for twelve weeks at a community retirement center in Athens, Georgia. Since the participants were volunteers, most were found to vary greatly, as they do in the general population. Among materials read were *Readers' Digest Magazine, Readers' Digest Condensed Novels, Time,* religious books, short stories, and a religious pamphlet. According to Wilson (1979), the few studies that have been done on the reading interests of adults indicate that interests are totally individualistic and that, furthermore, Readarama participants add credence to that statement.

While Wilson (1979) studied enhancing the lives of older adults through reading in retirement centers, Lovelace (1979) investigated the use of reading activities in the enhancement of the lives of nursing home patients. With reference to their interests, preliminary interviews with the director and the occupational therapist in a 100-bed convalescent home revealed that only 4 of the 100 patients appeared to read regularly materials other than the Bible and the newspaper. According to Lovelace (1979), the older adults like nostalgic stories, which provide a forum for reminiscing and discussion of the good old days. Lovelace (1979) found that while some patients browse through large-type editions of the *Reader's Digest,* little use was made of paperback novels placed in the patients' lounge. Although Talking Books were available, they were seldom used. At least these findings were true in this particular convalescent home. Lovelace (1979) attributes this lack of use of Talking Books to the fact that many of the residents were not readers prior to becoming visually or physically handicapped. Furthermore, she contends that the intellectual content of many of the titles as well as the prolonged attentiveness required may have lessened full enjoyment by the patient.

Gentile and McMillan (1979) sought to identify content that motivates the elderly to seek intellectual, physical, or spiritual renewal through reading-related exercises. Their central concern is with library experiences which elevate older people's values and attitudes, feelings of self-worth, sense of humor, and mental and physical development. Thus their concern is with encouraging them to revive dormant interests and explore new vistas in personal fulfillment. They provide a useful bibliotherapy of materials around the topical areas which they consider to be appropriate in reading programs for the aging, topics which appear to be centered around the theme of self-actualization.

With the limited information concerning the interests of older persons, it would be dangerous to generalize as to their interests. In light of the information available, it appears that their interests vary as widely as the readers themselves. Kingston (1979) notes that regardless of the reading interests, the aged, despite increased leisure time, do not develop reading habits unless they acquired them at an earlier age. No particular interest appears to be stereotypic of older adults, fortunately perhaps for the older adults, as they have been damaged too much already by being stereotyped by societal attitudes toward them.

Drickamer (1971) concluded that: people who read at an early age enjoy books more than those who had not read when they were younger; older adults do not enjoy fiction with confusing plots and many characters; large print and dull paper are preferred; and generally, depressing books, science fiction, and meditations are not enjoyed.

Nelson Associates (1969) found that older adults are not inclined toward how-to-do-it material, science fiction books, or books that are frank about sex or violence.

Furthermore, they have less need for vocational or professional reading material. However, there are, of course, exceptions to these findings and a wide range of reading material for older adults must be provided (Romani 1973).

With the present and ever-increasing numbers of older persons in the United States, combined with the limited information concerning their reading interests, it is apparent that further research into the interests of older adults is needed so that educational programs that enhance their lives and provide for self-actualization and self-fulfullment can be provided in ways such as the following: increased enjoyment of leisure time through reading; as an outlet and as a means for forming social contacts (Wilson 1979); as a means of renewal (Gentile and McMillan 1979); in enhancing the lives of the aging in retirement centers (Wilson 1979); and in enhancing the lives of nursing home patients (Lovelace 1979). Most people would agree that reading can enhance the life of anyone.

The major needs of older adults are usually identified as income maintenance, the preservation of physical and mental health, and finding a role in life. Consequently, efforts should be made to provide them with materials to keep them creative and functioning at their maximum capability (Romani 1973).

Typical of the national surveys is the one completed by Sharon (1973) in which he obtained information on the reading interests and habits of 5,067 adults throughout the country who were sixteen years of age or older. The period spent on various reading activities for this entire group was just under a daily average of two hours, while for those adults sixty years of age or older only eighty-nine minutes per day were devoted to reading-related activities. In summarizing the results of this study Sharon noted "young adults tend to read more than older persons, while the very old spend the least amount of time on reading" (p 158.).

In a similar study Pheiffer and Davis (1971) surveyed the leisure time reading activities of 502 adults aged 46-71. The results showed that the average weekly time spent on reading-related activities for the total group was approximately eighty-five hours with the women reading slightly more than the men. It was also found that the older members of this group spent significantly more time reading than did the younger readers.

There is strong evidence of the importance of reading in fulfilling needs of the older person for entertainment, knowledge, the satisfaction of intellectual curiosity, cultural development, and companionship—purposes not very different from that of any age group (Kanner 1972).

APPROACHES AND DELIVERY OF SERVICES

As mentioned earlier, bibliotherapy in its current form is used primarily as a group approach either in a development or clinical mode. The sharing of experiences through the identification or association of literary readings helps to bring about positive social-emotional development. Kingston (1973) has suggeted that reading in a social setting helps alleviate loneliness, relieves the pain of social deprivation, and reverses a decline of cognitive functioning resulting from a disuse of intellectual capability.

The Readarama Program

One such social-development approach, was conducted by Wilson (referred to earlier). Readarama was developed for a retirement center in Athens, Georgia. The publicly funded retirement center ran the program-study for twelve weeks in 1977. The following description details the essential elements, sequence of events, and results of the Readerama program.

Participants

Since Readarama was a voluntary program, the group members were all avid readers. The group, which included six regular participants and six others, bore out the finding of high educational levels for people interested in reading as a hobby. In addition, all members had been active, working women and were living in Athens to be near their children. The age range of the participants was fifty-nine to seventy-five. All viewed Readarama as a scheduled activity to look forward to each week.

No men participated in the group because Readarama conflicted with the very popular furniture-refinishing class at the center. Interestingly, most of the men at the center preferred more active classes rather than a reading group, though many were avid readers.

Reading Interests

The reading interests and habits of the members varied greatly, as they do in the general population. One member read *Readers' Digest* and *Readers' Digest Condensed Novels.* Another read *Time* and the newspaper. One woman, who was an insomniac, read and dozed all night. Her interest at present was in contemporary fiction, but she was an avid, lifelong reader, as were all of the participants.

Another member, who had recently lost two daughters in a car wreck, was reading a number of religious books, admittedly trying to understand their deaths. Another, who considered the group to be a class, reported on short stories from her grandaughter's high school literature books. A writer herself, she reported on the style and writing techniques of the authors and took notes on all the proceedings of Readarama sessions.

Still another member's reading interests were dictated by an unusual reading habit. She read a small religious pamphlet weekly because it was lightweight and she could lie in bed, flat on her back, and hold it up to read until she fell asleep. As she commented, "When I fall asleep and drop it, it won't wake me up."

Group Administration

While Readarama was a simply administered project, still several administrative problems deserve mention. First, Tuesday morning meetings proved to be somewhat of a problem because of the conflict with the furniture-refinishing class. Yet, this retirement center has such a comprehensive schedule that any other scheduled meeting time would have presented a conflict with some activity also. Certainly, a class for the elderly should be scheduled in the day, for few are willing to go out at night.

Second, because of complications in the mailing of the newsletters, the information on Readarama did not go out before the first scheduled meeting. Therefore, the retirement center director had to personally telephone interested people to publicize Readarama. The cooperation of the center director and staff added to the ease of runing the program.

Logistics problems arose, also, because the shuttle bus service provided to participants was often late in running. While these problems may have reduced the number of participants, it also insured that all participants were avid readers and interested in participating in the group.

Group Organization

Since no literature was available on how to set up this type of group, the organization was very flexible initially. Because no precedent was available, the leader decided to provide a story for everyone to read at the first session in order to generate discussion. Attending members chose to follow along as the group leader read an article on Truman aloud rather than volunteering to read aloud themselves or to read silently. It was immediately apparent by their restlessness and boredom that this read-aloud method would not be acceptable on a weekly basis. This could have been anticipated since all were good readers themselves.

They began the discussion by saying they did not remember Truman, but by the end of the first session, members decided they not only remembered Truman but wanted to discuss him further the following week. Before the next meeting everyone had individually read something about Truman or the Carter election, which also became part of the conversation.

It is to be noted that many stimulating discussions in the twelve weeks were prefaced by "I don't remember." Anyone planning a group of this type must be careful to be optimistic and provide probes to memory without being forceful and pushy.

Readarama members agreed on group policy during the second meeting. Everyone would read something during the week independently, and the Readarama time would be used to discuss the individual reading and to exchange book ideas. By this point in time, both the members and the leader recognized that vast differences in reading interests and the amount members could read during the week would require a flexible group procedure. Conducting the class by group decision was very important to the members. They were alert to avoiding a class where the leader taught, bossed, and forced people to read aloud or made assignments.

The leader voluntarily supplied a story each week, which members took home to read if they wanted to. The story was strictly supplementary, not assigned reading. All stories were taken from *Seventy Most Unforgettable Characters from Readers' Digest* (1967). The preferences for the ten *Readers' Digest* stories, all short biographies, show a certain pattern that should be noted. The two most popular stories used were "Angel from Maine" by Robert P. Tristam Coffin about a woman raising her family in the frontier islands of Maine and "Country Doctor" by Helen Graham Rezatto about a midwestern doctor. Both were set in the early 1900s and were reminiscent of the participants' early childhood days. In contrast, the least favorite story of those used was "Unforgettable Benchley" by Marc Connelly about the work and life of Robert Benchley. It was a factual account of Benchley's life. Other similarly factual stories were less preferred also.

While preferences were stated, all participants indicated that they had read the story weekly no matter what it was or how well they liked it. When they missed a session, they asked for copies of the story missed. The *Readers' Digest* stories were passed on to other nongroup members also. Most participants stated that they enjoyed the stories because they were short and entertaining.

Group Discussions

The Readarama sessions generated discussion not only of reading and books but also of life reminiscences and social problems. Readarama participants were much too busy to read for long periods of time except as a means of overcoming insomnia. All participants read the newspaper daily and seemed to dismiss that as not really reading. Magazines were not read, because they were considered to be too expensive. Book choices mentioned by members showed a preference for short stories or condensations of historical novels. The participants did not buy books because of the expense. Instead, they were given books and swapped them with neighbors, friends, and their children. Only one used the public library; others said it was inaccessible.

In group sessions, each member reported on her reading in turn. While the members had expressed interest in exchanging book ideas, none indicated overwhelming interest in reading what anyone else had read. There was never any mention made of reading what someone else had suggested. Primarily each member read in her own interest area throughout the course of Readarama. Each person reported her reading, the group generated discussion on the topic, and went on to the next topic. At first the leader tried to read and join in the discussion, but it was apparent that the members considered her a listener not a participant.

The talk stimulated during the discussions was as interesting as the reports on the reading. The recurrent topics were the current state of the world, including Carter's presidency, the energy crisis, and violence. Violence with children was a surprisingly recurrent theme in the discussions. All the women were concerned with child abuse as well as the violence that children see on television.

Results

Several comments can be made about the Readarama programs. First, the ladies in the group did not have time to read a great deal. They read like the rest of the active adults are perceived to read, a bit here and a bit there. Second, the group was a means of getting together with other readers for a social hour. It was a social outlet and a way for previously active adults to maintain some level of activity and structure in their retired lives. Third, the reminiscences stemming from reading and discussion were the most enjoyable part of the group for all participants. The ladies enjoyed sharing memories of their early married lives and enjoyed explain things to the young leader who was treated as a granddaughter. Yet, their interests in current events showed them to still be active members of society as well.

The actual reading interests of the participants were varied to such a great degree that any regimentation of the group would have been impossible. It is noted that any reading group for healthy and active aged persons would have to be run either as a class (which this group did not want) or would have to be very open and unstructured, as this group was. No requirements were put on group members in Readarama whatever. The few times the leader tried to create structure, participants balked and stated emphatically that they were not in school anymore.

Community problems raised during group interactions showed the group to be engaged and very interested in society and current events. They felt that the elderly could give valuable insight to the younger generation on some of today's social problems. However, they felt that young people were not willing to listen to them or their advice.

Other Examples

Before bibliotherapy can be implemented, obstacles preventing the delivery of literary materials to the aging must be removed. While library sites may logically serve the needs of the healthy aging population, different strategies are necessary for the infirmed, hospitalized, and residents of nursing and retirement homes. Reed (1973) has identified a variety of resource strategies throughout the country. The bookmobile is one means through which services can be provided to the aging. A bookmobile which provides direct service to various institutions and neighborhoods in Milwaukee where concentrations of the elderly live is equipped with a hydraulic lift, which makes it possible for people in wheelchairs to enter it. The South of Market Area Demonstration in San Francisco has a multi-media van which takes taped programs and films as well as books into the downtown area it serves, where many isolated old people live. A "MultiMedia Mobile" is constructed for the Daniel Boone Regional Library in Missouri, to serve isolated people of all ages in a predominantly rural area. It is equipped with a 16mm projection system, front and rear projection screens, a 35mm filmstrip/players and a listening system, display areas, a puppet stage, demonstrations of various types of reading aids for the visually handicapped, and puppet shows which will appeal to old people as well as the children.

A carefully planned shut-in service for individual home delivery has been incorporated into the Toronto Public Library's Traveling Branch, which already offered service with book deposits in homes and clubs for the aged, and bedside booktruck service in hospitals. They use a station wagon for this service, and have found no need for special equipment other than heavy webbing straps to bundle together the books for each borrower. They have also found useful what they call a "bundlebuggy" for use in apartment houses, especially those for the elderly where several borrowers live in a building. An intensive publicity campaign preceded the initiation of the service, which is limited to genuine shut-ins. Some elderly people are eligible only in the winter! They note that the general reading level for users of this service is higher than in institutions for the elderly, and believe this is because the people who can remain in their own homes are likely to be in more active physical conditon.

In some instances the aging are brought to the library rather than taking the library to them. The Madison Heights Public Library in Michigan busses senior citizens to the libary where special programs, such as handicraft demonstations, book reviews and discussions, are scheduled for them. The library began the service on a three-day-a-week basis with a rented bus; it proved so satisfactory that the schedule is being expanded with a bus purchased by the library.

In North Dakota, one library uses a Volkswagen bus to bring senior citizens into the library on a regular schedule; another uses what it calls "The Free Wheeler" to transport the elderly from rest homes and housing units to the library; still another pays fare to and from the library. While not intended specifically for the aging, the arrangement by which the Marion Public Library in Indiana has reimbursed the city-owned bus company for each one-way ticket used by a library patron has been of special benefit to older people. The librarian points out that "Many passengers are retired persons whose income is limited; reading is a favorite pastime with them and they come often."

A combination of outreach and in-library service for the aging is found in Newton, Massachusetts in the "drop-in center." One drop-in center, in a branch library, is "open eight hours a day with comfortable furniture, a continuous coffee-pot, reading material, games, etc., for the senior citizens to enjoy." The library conducts book-talk-coffee hours at apartments for the elderly, and also, by invitation, at drop-in centers in local churches. A service which includes many elderly people, the Center for the Visually Handicapped in the Newton Free Library, is "based on a philosophic conviction that visually handicapped persons must not be separated from, but rather, encouraged to use public library resources and facilities." The same philosophic base regarding the aging apparently underlies the programs planned specifically for them in this library.

The kinds of special equipment available, often for loan, have been greatly expanded in recent years. There are magnifiers, large print typewriters and Braillers, special games and playing cards for the visually handicapped, bed specs and ceiling projectors for bedridden patients, photocopying equipment, and stands for large print books, as well as the specially equipped mobile units mentioned earlier.

FUTURE TRENDS

Bibliotherapy can be used by therapists (facilitators), educators, librarians, and other qualified personnel in the health professions. Community agencies, who have qualified staff, can give the aging a chance to discuss their reactions to issues in a personalized manner. Through identifying with a character in a book or reacting to a situation in a film, people can discuss themselves in a nonthreatening atmosphere due to the objectivity which literature provides. As Shrodes (1950) explained it: "Literature brings at once a fantasy and yet a realistic portrayal of human behavior, permits the reader, paradoxically, both an illusion of psychic distance and immediacy of experience." Therefore, bibliotherapy can be a group awareness method both for people to talk about themselves and for people who need the distance afforded by literature.

With regard to the field of "reading" as it relates to the aging, many questions remain unanswered. Research, done primarily through surveys, has not provided a sufficient and clear enough understanding of the effects of reading upon the aging. Further research in this area is necessary. Robinson (1976) developed a list of ready research areas using the elderly as a population that have not been developed. They are the following:

1. etiology and characteristics of avid and mature aged readers
2. flexibility (rate and comprehension) of reading behaviors on the part of aged persons
3. construction and validation of instruments designed to assess the reading competency and maturity of aged persons
4. effects of bibliotherapy for the aging
5. usefulness of readability formulae in recommending reading to aged individuals
6. relationship between listening comprehension and reading comprehension in aged persons
7. relationships between the self-concepts of the aging and their reading behavior
8. critical and creative reading behaviors of the aging
9. effectiveness and value of individualized reading programs versus group programs for aged persons
10. validity and usefulness of close, informal reading inventories, and standardized reading tests for the aging
11. relationships between oral language performance of aged persons and their reading performance
12. reading behaviors of important groups of aged persons, for

example, the intellectually gifted, cultural minorities
13. evaluation of reading programs for the elderly in institutions and for those living outside of institutions
14. assessment of reading needs of the elderly as well as asessment of their interests
15. effects of large-print books, talking books, and other technical devices on the reading behavior of the elderly
16. effect of societal expectations of the abilities of the elderly on their reading behaviors and interests

In conclusion, it may be worthy to draw attention to the research of Frenkel-Brunswick (1968) who noted that numerous anatomical processes are influenced by one's inner life, such as knowledge and experience, and actually impeded biological decline. If this is true, reading and writing pursuits deserve high priority among the aged. It becomes imperative for older adults to vigorously combat the ennui that oozes into their daily lives, calling on them to quit, passively watch TV, or putter at some meaningless task. They must awaken to the fact that more, rather than less, knowledge and experience represent the only way out of their current dilemma. Their emotional, psychic, spiritual, and corporeal energy may be rekindled through the avenues of literary enterprise, thereby opening an aperature to a significant future.

References

Ansello, E. F. Age and ageism in children's first literature. *Educational Gerontology,* 1977, 255-274.

Berry, F. Toward a research basis for the distinction between educational/humanistic and clinical modes of bibliotherapy. In *Seminar on Bibliotherapy.* Madison, University of Wisconsin Library School. 1978.

De Santi, R. J., The older reader: an investigation of the reading strategies, habits, and interests of four persons sixty years of age or older. (Doctoral dissertation, Indiana University, 1976). *Dissertation Abstracts International,* 1976, *37,* 4719A (University Microfilms No. 77-3285)

Drickamer, J. Rhode Island project: book reviews by older citizens. *Library Journal,* 1971:2737-2748.

Eklund, L. Aging and the field of education. In M. W. Riley, J. W. Riley, Jr., & M. E. Johnson (eds.), *Aging and society: aging and the professions. New York: Russell Sage Foundation,* 1969: 328-329.

Frenkel-Brunswick, E. Adjustments and reorientations in the course of the life span. In B. Neugarten (ed.), *Middle age and aging,* pp. 74-84.Chicago, IL: University of Chicago Press, 1968.

Gentile, L. M., & McMillan, M. Reading: a means of renewal for the aged. *Educational Gerontology,* 1979, *4:* 215-222.

Hannigan, Margaret C. The librarian in bibliotherapy: pharmacist or bibliotherapist?'' *Library Trends,* October 1962: 192.

Kingston, A. J., Jr. Areas of concern about reading. In P. Nacke (ed.),*Programs & practices for college reading (Vol. 2), 22nd yearbook of the National Reading Conference,* p. 53-56, Boone, NC: National Reading Conference, 1973.

Kingston, A. J., Jr., Reading and the aged: a statement of the problem. *Educational Gerontology,* 1979, *4:* 205-207.

Lovelace, T. Reading activities to enhance the lives of nursing home patients. *Educational Gerontology,* 1979, *4:* 239-243.

Monroe, M. E. Reader services and bibliotherapy. In M. Monroe, (ed.) *Reading guidance and bibliotherapy in public, hospital and institutional libraries,* pp. 40-44. Madison, University of Wisconsin Library School, 1971.

Moshey, K. M. The retired adult reader: his reading interests and choices and the readability levels of them. Master of Education thesis, Rutgers University, 1972.

Nelson Associates, U.S. Library of Congress, Division for the Blind and Physically Handicapped. A survey of reading interests and equipment preferences. A study of circulation systems in selected regional libraries. Washington, D.C.: Nelson Associates, 1969, vi.

Pheiffer, E., & Davis, G. L. The use of leisure time in middle life. *The Gerontologist,* 1971, *11:* 187-195.

Reed, E. Library programs and activities: serving the aging directly. *Library Trends,* January, *1973:* 404-412.

Riley, M. W., & Foner, A. *Aging society: an inventory of research findings.* New York: Russell Sage Foundation, 1968, 1, 512.

Robinson, R. D., & Maring, G. The aging process and its relationship to reading. A review of the literature from gerontology with implications for future research in reflections and investigations in reading. In G. McVinch & W. Miller (eds.), *Reflections and investigations on reading.* pp. 870-878. Clemson, SC: National Reading Conference, 25th Yearbook, 1976.

Romani, D. Reading needs and interests of older people. *Library Trends,* 1973, *21:* 390-403.

Rubin, Rhea J. *Using bibliotherapy: a guide to theory and practice.* Phoenix, Oryx Press, 1978.

Sharon, A. T. What Do Adults Read? *Reading Research Quarterly,* 1973-1974, *9:* 148-169.

Tews, Ruth M. Introduction. *Library Trends,* October, 1962, *99.*

Tuckman, J. and Lorge, I. ''The influence of a course on the psychology of adults on attitudes toward old people and older workers. *Journal of Educational Psychology,* 1952: 400-407.

Wilson, J. M. Enhancing the lives of the aged in a retirement center through a program of reading. *Educational Gerontology,* 1979, *4:* 245-251

Poetry Therapy Readings

Anonymous. Poetry therapy. *Time,* March 13, 1972, *45.*

Anonymous. Poetry therapy: an idea whose time has come. *Roche Report,* April 1, 1970.

Anonymous. P. T. gets new meaning: poetry therapy. *American Journal of Nursing,* 1972, *72,*: 1034.

Abbe, G. Poetry, the great therapy: a statement of faith. American Weise Whetstone Publishers, n.d.

Abrams, A. S. Poetry therapy in the psychiatric hospital. In Arthur Lerner (ed.), *Poetry in the therapeutic experience,* pp. 63-71. New York: Pergamon, 1978.

Anderson, C. J. Poetry Therapy in Psychiatric Nursing. Paper presented at the General Council Meeting of the International Federation of Library Associations (40th, Wash., D.C., Nov. 16-23, 1974). (ERIC document ED 104 453).

Anderson, C. J. Poetry therapy in psychiatric nursing. *Libri* (Copenhagen), 1975, *25:* 133-37.

Andrews, M. Poetry programs in mental hospitals. *Perspectives in Psychiatric Care,* 1975, *13,:* 17-18.

Baldwin, N. The therapeutic implications of poetry writing: a methodology. *Journal of Psychedelic Drugs,* 1976, *8:* 307-12.

Berkley, B. J. Poetry in a cage: therapy in a correctional setting. In Jack J. Leedy (ed.), *Poetry the Healer,* pp. 1-16. Philadelphia; Lippincott, 1973.

Barron, J. Poetry and therapeutic communication: nature and meaning of poetry. *Psychotherapy: Theory, Research and Practice,* 1974, *11:* 87-92.

Becker, B. J. Insightful verses. *American Journal of Psychoanalysis,* 1971, *31:* 103.

Berger, A. Festival of poetry therapy at UCLA. *Los Angeles Weekley News,* Dec. 21-28, 1973: 3-4.

Berger, A. Self-discovery for teacher and youngster through poetry. In Jack J. Leedy (ed.), *Poetry the healer,* pp. 175-96. Philadelphia: Lippincott, 1973.

Berger, M. Poetry as therapy—and therapy as poetry. In Jack J. Leedy (ed.), *Poetry therapy. . . ,* pp. 75-87. Philadelphia: Lippincott, 1969.

Berry, F. M. Approaching poetry therapy from a scientific orientation. In Arthur Lerner (ed.), *Poetry in the therapeutic experience,* pp. 127-42. New York: Pergamon, 1978.

Blanton, S. *The healing power of poetry.* New York: Crowell, 1960

Blanton, S. The Use of Poetry in Individual Psychotherapy. In Jack J. Leedy (ed.), *Poetry Therapy. . . ,* pp. 171-79.

Blinderman, A. Shamans, witch doctors, medicine men and poetry. In Jack J. Leedy (ed.), *Poetry the healer.* Philadelphia: Lippincott, 1973. pp. 127-41.

Brothers, B. Psychotherapy and the fine arts and me. *Voices: Journal of the American Academy of Psychotherapists,* Winter, 1975-76, *11:* 66-68.

Buck, L., and A. Kramer. Opening new worlds to the deaf and the disturbed. In Jack. J. Leedy (ed.), *Poetry the healer,* pp. 142-74. Philadelphia: Lippincott, 1973.

Buck, L, and A. Kramer. Poetry as a means of group facilitation. *Journal of Humanistic Psychology,* Winter, 1974, *14:* 57-71.

Burke, K., Thoughts on the poets' corner. In Jack J. Leedy (ed.), *Poetry Therapy. . . ,* Philadelphia: Lippincott, 1969

Cahn, M. Poetic Dimensions of Encounter. In Arthur Burton (ed.), *Encounter: The theory and practice of encounter groups,* pp. 97-111. San Francisco: Jossey-Bass, 1969.

Card, P. Poetry as a bridge to the lost. *RN,* March 1969, *32:* 46-49.

Chaliff, C. Emily Dickinson and poetry therapy: the art of peace. In Jack J. Leedy (ed.), *Poetry the healer,* pp. 24-49. Philadelphia: Lippincott, 1973.

Chase, J. Poems struggling to be born. *Human Behavior,* Aug., 1973, *2,* 24-49. (Reprinted, as by Janet Chase-Marshall, in Walt Anderson (ed.), *Therapy and the arts: tools of consciousness,* pp. 79-89. New York: Harper and Row [Colophon paperback], 1977.

Clancy, M. and R. Lauer. Zen telegrams: a warm-up technique for poetry therapy groups. In Arthur Lerner (ed.), *Poetry in the Therapeutic Experience,* pp. 97-107. New York: Pergamon, 1978.

Coogan, J. P. Apollo and Psyche—poetry as therapy. *SK&F Psychiatric Reporter,* Sept.-Oct., 1966, *28,* 20-23. Smith, Kline & French Laboratories; 1500 Spring Garden Street; Philadelphia, PA 19101.

Crootof, C. Poetry therapy for psychoneurotics in a mental health center. In Jack J. Leedy (ed.), *Poetry therapy. . .,* pp. 38-51. Philadelphia: Lippincott, 1969.

Davis, L. The paraprofessional and poetry therapy. In Arthur Lerner (ed.), *Poetry in the therapeutic experience,* pp. 108-13. New York: Pergamon, 1978.

Edgar, K. The epiphany of the self via poetry therapy. In Arthur Lerner (ed.), *Poetry in the therapeutic experience,* pp. 24-40. New York: Pergamon, 1978.

Edgar, K., and R. Hazley. A curriculum proposal for training poetry therapists. In Jack J. Leedy (ed.), *Poetry Therapy. . .,* pp. 260-268. Philadelphia: Lippincott, 1969.

Edgar, K., and R. Hazley. Validation of poetry therapy as a group therapy technique. In Jack J. Leedy (ed.), *Poetry Therapy. . .,* pp. 111-23. Philadelphia: Lippincott, 1969.

Edgar, K., R. Hazley, and Herbert I. Levit. Poetry therapy with hospitalized schizophrenics. In Jack J. Leedy, (ed.), *Poetry Therapy.,* pp. 29-37. Philadelphia: Lippincott, 1969.

Ellis, L. B., and F. M. Berry. A partial listing of sources related to bibliotherapy and poetry therapy: a second run at a comprehensive listing. (Mimeograph), 1976. pp. 64.

Erikson, C. R., and R. Lejeune. Poetry as a subtle therapy. *Hospital and Community Psychiatry.* Feb., 1972, *23,* 56-57.

Evans, R. V. Poetry therapy. Paper presented at the Anniversary of the Florida Council of Teachers of English State Conference (50th, Daytona Beach, Fl. Oct. 17-19, 1974). (ERIC document ED 099 868).

Favardin, P. *From poetry to poetry therapy.* (Translated title of a book in Persian; author's address: 145 Pahlavi Ave.; Amir Akram Square; Tehran, Iran.)

Fine, H. J., Howard R. Pollio, and Charles H. Simpkinson. Figurative language metaphor and psychotherapy. *Psychotherapy: theory, research, and practice,* 1973, *10,* 87-91.

Fitzgibbon, C. Poetry and interpersonal communication. *Volta Review,* Jan., 1971, *73,* 58-59

Forrest, D. V. The patient's sense of the poem: affinities and ambiguities. In Jack

J. Leedy (ed.), *Poetry therapy...*, pp. 231-59. Philadelphia: Lippincott, 1969.

Gelberman, J. H., and D. Kobak. The psalms as psychological and allegorical poems: therapeutic applications in a clinical setting. In Jack J. Leedy (ed.), *Poetry therapy...*, pp. 133-41. Philadelphia, Lippincott, 1969.

Goldfield, M. D., and R. M. Lauer. The use of creative writing in groups of young drug abusers. *The New Physician.* July, 1971: 449-57.

Greenberg, S. A. Poetry therapy in a self-help group: AFTLI and/or poetry therapy. In Jack J. Leedy (ed.), *Poetry therapy...*, pp. 212-22. Philadelphia: Lippincott, 1969. (Author is founder of AFTLI—Association for Feeling Truth and Living It.)

Greenwald, H. Poetry as communication in psychotherapy. In Jack J. Leedy (ed.), *Poetry Therapy...*, pp. 142-54. Philadelphia: Lippincott, 1969.

Greifer, E. Poetry Therapy. *The Brooklyn Psychologist,* Sept., 1964.

Greifer, E. *Principles of poetry therapy.* New York: Poetry Therapy Center, 1963.

Hamilton, J. W. Gender rejection as a reaction to early sexual trauma and its partial expression in verse. *British Journal of Medical Psychology,* 1968, *41:* 405-10.

Harari, C. (See Molly Harrower).

Harrower, M. Poems emerging from the therapeutic experience. *Journal of Nervous and Mental Disease,* 1969, *149:* 213-23.

Harrower, M. *The therapy of poetry.* Springfield, Illionois: Charles C. Thomas, 1972. (Autobiographical account, from childhood.)

Harrower, M. "The therapy of poetry." In Jules Masserman (ed.), *Current Psychiatric Therapies,* Vol. 14, pp. 97-105. New York: Grune & Stratton, 1974.

Harrower, M. Variations on the theme: artist as therapist, therapist as artist. *Voices: Journal of the American Academy of Psychotherapists,* Winter, 1975-76, *11:* 5-9.

Harrower, M. Charles Crootof, Rolland Parker, and Carmi Harari. Poetry as therapy and therapist as poet. *Journal of Clinical Issues in Psychology,* May, 1970, *1:* 34-38.

Hayakawa, S. I. Postscript: metamessages and self-discovery. In Jack J. Leedy (ed.), *Poetry Therapy...*, pp. 269-72. Philadelphia: Lippincott, 1969.

Heninger, O. E. Poetry therapy in private practice: an odyssey into the healing power of poetry. In Arthur Lerner (ed.), *Poetry in the therapeutic experience,* pp. 56-62. New York: Pergamon, 1978.

Hitchings, W. D. Poetry, a way to fuller awareness: added dimension in treating addicts. In Jack J. Leedy (ed.), *Poetry therapy...*, pp. 124-32. Philadelphia, Lippincott, 1969.

Hunsiger, P. *The educational uses of poetry therapy.* 1976. 23 pp. (ERIC document ED 130, 373).

Jarrell, R. *The bat-poet.* Pictures by Maurice Sendak. New York: Macmillan; London: Collier-Macmillan, 1963. (Ostensibly a book for children, it is also about poetry and poets, and, in places, about poetry therapy—minus the label.)

Jones, L. A poet-in-residence at a mental hospital. *LA Magazine,* July 29, 1972: 29. (On Dr. Arthur Lerner.)

Jones, R. E. The double door: poetry therapy for adolescents. In Jack J. Leedy (ed.), *Poetry therapy...*, pp. 223-30. Philadelphia: Lippincott, 1969.

Jones, R. E. Treatment of a psychotic patient by poetry therapy, with a historical

note. In Jack J. Leedy (ed.), *Poetry therapy. . .*, pp. 19-28. Philadelphia, Lippincott, 1969.

Kaplan, J. "Poetry therapy"—new and for mental illness. *Seventeen.* Jan. 1973,
32: 28.

Kobak, D. Poetry therapy in a "600" school and in a counseling center: creative
writing as a therapeutic instrument. In Jack J. Leedy (ed.), *Poetry Therapy. . .*,
pp. 180-87. Philadelphia: Lippincott, 1969.

Kobak, D., and E. Nisenson. Poetry therapy: A Way to Solve Emotional
Problems." *Instructor,* Dec., 1971, *81:* 76-77.

Koslow, S. P. Poetry Therapy. *Mademoiselle,* March, 1972, *74:* 48.

Kramer, A. The Use of Poetry in a Private Mental Hospital. In Jack J. Leedy
(ed.), *Poetry therapy. . .*, pp. 200-11. Philadelphia: Lippincott, 1969.

La Rue, L. There's no rhyme or reason, but poetry-therapy works! Long Beach
[CA] *Independent Press-Telegram,* Nov. 4, 1978, b: 1-2.

Lauer, R. Abuses of poetry therapy. In Arthur Lerner (ed.), *Poetry in the Therapeutic experience,* pp. 72-80. New York: Pergamon, 1978.

Lauer, R. Creative writing as therapeutic tool. *Hospital and Community Psychiatry,*
Feb., 1972, *23:* 55-56.

Lauer, R. and M. Goldfield. Creative writing in group therapy. *Psychotherapy,* 1970
7, 248-52.

Lawler, J. Poetry Therapy? *Psychiatry,* 1972, *35:* 227-37.

Leedy, J. J. Poetry and medicine. *MD: Medical Newsmagazine,* July, 1964, *3.*

Leedy, J. J. *Poetry therapy: a new ancillary therapy in psychiatry.* New York: Poetry
Therapy Center, 1966.

Leedy, J., ed. *Poetry therapy: the use of poetry in the treatment of emotional disorders.*
Philadelphia: Lippincott, 1969.

Leedy, J. J. Principles of poetry therapy. In Jack J. Leedy (ed.), *Poetry Therapy. . .*,
pp. 67-74. Philadelphia: Lippincott, 1969.

Leedy, J. J., ed. *Poetry the healer.* Philadelphia: Lippincott, 1973.

Leedy, J. J., The value of poetry therapy. *American Journal of Psychiatry,* 1970,
126: 1183-84. (Letter.)

Leedy, J. J., and Elaine Rapp. Poetry therapy and some links to art therapy.
Art Psychotherapy, 1973, *1:* 145-51.

Lerner, A. Poetry therapy and a "freedom to move in any direction." *Showcase,*
magazine of the Chicago Sun-Times, Sunday July 16, 1972, *2.*

Lerner, A. Poetry therapy: from sad to verse. *PTA Magazine,* March 1973, *67,*
30-32: 36-37.

Lerner, A. Poetry therapy. *American Journal of Nursing,* 1973, *73:* 1336-38.

Lerner, A. Poetry therapy: a healing art. *The Study of English,* Tokyo, 1974.

Lerner, A. Poetry as therapy. *APA Monitor,* Sept.-Oct., 1975: *6,* 4.

Lerner, A. Entries from a journal on poetry and therapy. *Voices: Journal of the
American Academy of Psychotherapists,* Winter, 1975-76, *11:* 60-71.

Lerner, A. A look at poetry therapy. *Art Psychotherapy,* 1976, *3:* i-ii.

Lerner, A. ed. *Poetry in the therapeutic experience.* New York: Pergamon Press, 1978.
(Also see interview, under Shiffrin.)

Lessner, J. W. The poem as catalyst in group counseling. *The Personnel and Guidance
Journal,* Sept., 1974, *53:* 33-38.

McDaniel, C. G. Sartre, Salinger, and psychotherapy. Riverside [CA] *Press,* Mon., July 9, 1973, A-8 (AP wire service story on use of literature—esp.poetry—in Northwestern University Medical School therapy program.)

Marlin, W. A portrait through poetry and drawing. *American Journal of Art Therapy,* April, 1974, 13: 237-249. (Case study of 39-yr.-old cancer patient attempting to deal with her emotional problems through her poetry and drawings.)

Maycock, T. The Muse as a psychotherapist. *The New York Times,* Sunday, April 30, 1972, *1:1:* 15-16.

Meerlo, J. A. M. The universal language of rhythm. In Jack J. Leedy (ed.), *Poetry Therapy. . . ,* pp. 52-66. Philadelphia: Lippincott, 1969.

Miller, A. H. The spontaneous use of poetry in an adolescent girls' group. *International Journal of Group Psychotherapy,* 1973, *23.* 223-227.

Morrison, M. R. Poetry therapy with disturbed adolescents: bright arrows on a dark river. In Jack J. Leedy, (ed.), *Poetry therapy. . . ,* pp. 88-103. Philadelphia: Lippincott, 1969.

Morrison, M. R. A defense of poetry therapy. In Jack J. Leedy (ed.), *Poetry the Healer,* pp. 77-90. Philadelphia: Lippincott, 1973.

Murphy, J. M. Foreword to Jack J. Leedy (ed.), *Poetry the healer,* pp. ix-xvi. Lippincott, 1973.

Nemiah, J. C. The art of deep thinking: reflections on poetry and psychotherapy. *Seminars in Psychiatry,* 1973, *5:* 301-311.

Parker, R. S. Poetry as a therapeutic art—in the resolution of resistance in psychotherapy. In Jack J. Leedy (ed.), *Poetry therapy. . . ,* pp. 155-70. Philadelphia: Lippincott, 1969.

Pattison, E. M. The psychodynamics of poetry by patients. In Jack J. Leedy (ed.), *Poetry the healer,* pp. 197-214, Philadelphia: Lippincott, 1973.

Pietropinto, A. Exploring the unconscious through nonsense poetry. In Jack J. Leedy (ed.), *Poetry the healer,* pp. 50-76. Philadelphia: Lippincott, 1973.

Putzel, J. Toward alternative theories of poetry therapy. Ed.D. dissertation, University of Massachusetts, 1975. (Abstract in *Dissertation Abstracts International,* 1975, *36:* 3012b-13b.)

Rance, C., and A. Price. Poetry as a group project. *American Journal of Occupational Therapy,* 1973, *27:* 252-55. (Rationale and procedures of such a group in a psychiatric setting.)

Reiter, S. The future of poetry therapy. *Art Psychotherapy,* 1978 *5:* 13-14.

Robinson, S. S., and J. K. Mowbray. Why poetry? In Jack J. Leedy (ed.), *Poetry therapy.,* pp. 188-99.

Rosenbaum, J. B. Review of Jack J. Leedy, ed. *Poetry therapy: the use of poetry in the treatment of emotional disorders. American Journal of Psychiatry,* 1969. *126:* 425.

Ross, D. L. Poetry therapy versus traditional supportive therapy: a comparison of group process. Ph.D. dissertation, Case Western Reserve University 1977. (Abstract in *Dissertation Abstracts International,* 1977, 38: 1417b-18b.)

Ross, R. N. Unlocking the doors of perception: poetry the healer. *Psychotherapy: Theory, Research and Practice,* 1975, *12:* 255-57. (Review-article on Jack J. Leedy, ed. *Poetry the healer.*)

Ross, R. N. Parsing concepts: a discovery technique for poetry therapy.: In Arthur Lerner (ed.), *Poetry in the therapeutic experience,* pp. 41-55. New York: Pergamon, 1978.

Rothenberg, A. Poetry in therapy, therapy in poetry. *The Sciences,* Jan.-Feb., 1972, *4:* 30-31.

Rothenberg, A. Poetic Process and psychotherapy. *Psychiatry,* 1972, 35: 238-54.

Rothenberg, A. Poetry and psychotherapy: kinships and contrasts, In Jack J. Leedy (ed.), *Poetry the healer,* pp. 91-126. Philadelphia: Lippincott, 1973.

Sansweet, S. J. In poetry, there could be reason as well as rhyme. Some therapists use poems as a way to aid patients; ulcer or an incipient poem?'' *The Wall Street Journal,* Pacific Coast Edition, March 13, 1975, 1d, 18c.

Schecter, R. L. Poetry: a therapeutic tool in the treatment of drug abuse. In Jack J. Leedy (ed.), *Poetry the Healer,* pp. 17-23. Philadelphia: Lippincott, 1973.

Schloss, G. A. *Psychopoetry: a new approach to self-awareness through poetry therapy.* New York: Grosset and Dunlap, 1976.

Schloss, G. A., and D. E. Grundy. Poetry therapy. *Literature & Psychology,* 1971, *21:* 51-55.

Schloss, G. A., and D. E. Grundy. Action techniques in psychopoetry. In Arthur Lerner (ed.), *Poetry in the therapeutic experience,* pp. 81-96. New York: Pergamon, 1978.

Sheff, E. T. Poetry as therapy—pathway to self discovery. M. S. degree project, California State University, Long Beach, 1977. (Abstract in *Masters Abstracts,* 1977, *15:* 117-18.)

Shiffrin, N. An interview with Dr. Arthur Lerner. *Stonecloud,* 1973 *2:* 13-16.

Silverman, H. L. Psychological implications of poetry therapy. *Society and Culture,* 1973, *4:* 215-28.

Solomon, J. Poetry therapy. *The Sciences,* Jan.-Feb., 1972, *12:* 20-25.

Sonne, J. C. Metaphors and Relationships. *Family Process,* 1964, *3:* 425-27.

Spector, S. I. Poetry therapy. *Voices: The Art & Science of Psychotherapy,* Winter, 1968, *4:* 31-40.

Stainbrook, E. Poetry and behavior in the psychotherapeutic experience. In Arthur Lerner (ed.), *Poetry in the therapeutic experience,* pp. 1-11. New York: Pergamon, 1978.

Weinstock, D. J., Poetry and the self. *CCEE Newsletter,* March, 1977: 10-19. (California Conference on English Education) (Abridged version of item 125.)

Weinstock, D. J. Poetry and the self: A brief autobiographical overview of some successes and some flops using 'poetry therapy' techniques in conventional and experimental classes, with implications for english teachers anywhere. ERIC Clearinghouse on Reading and Communication Skills, 1979. (Originally given as a paper at the 1977 meeting of the California Association of Teachers of English.)

Weinstock, D. J. Poetry therapy: a bibliography. (Mimeographed) 1979.

Wescott, R. W. The antiquity and universality of poetry therapy. *Scimitar and Song* (Edgewater, MD), March, 1972, *34:* 14.

White, G. The healing muse. *SK&F Psychiatric Reporter,* May-June, 1964, 14: 11-13. (Smith, Kline & French Laboratories; 1500 Spring Garden Street; Philadelphia, PA 19101.)

Wood, J. C. An experience in poetry therapy *Journal of Psychiatric Nursing and Mental Health Services,* 1975, *13,* 27-31.

Wood, J. C. Poetry threapy. In Mark Bricklin (ed.), *The Practical Encyclopedia of Natural Healing.* Emmaus, PA: Rodale, 1976. pp. 418-23. (Excerpted from item 129.)

7
Behavior Therapy with the Aging

Marian L. MacDonald
Bruce B. Kerr

Behavior therapy is a relatively recent addition to the knowledge base of the helping professions. Perhaps because of its newness, behavior therapy is sometimes misunderstood, at times even by therapists whose aim is to use it for therapeutic benefit (Kazdin 1980). Done correctly, however, behavioral interventions are demonstrably effective for treating many types of psychological problems; in some cases, they have been found to be effective where all other treatments have failed (Redd, Porterfield, and Andersen 1979; Ullman and Krasner 1965, 1974; Wilson and O'Leary 1980).

Several features of behavior therapy in addition to its effectiveness—including its emphasis on the present rather than the past, its quickness to produce noticeable behavior change, and its suitability for use by supervised paraprofessionals—make it a particularly valuable approach for work with the aging. This chapter is intended as an introduction in that context; it provides a brief overview of the history and current status of behavior therapy as well as a selective survey of some behavioral interventions with aging persons.

THE HISTORY AND CURRENT STATUS OF BEHAVIOR THERAPY

During the 1950's, a number of clinical psychologists became disenchanted with traditional psychotherapies because of their failure to produce client behavior change. They began looking for alternative treatments and were intrigued by the laboratory results of their academic colleagues studying learning. Their interest in exploring what would happen if the principles of learning found in the laboratory were applied to the behavior problems found in their clients gave rise to what was later called the behavioral movement (Ullmann 1969).

From these origins, however, the field of behavior therapy has not developed into a monolithic approach to problems in living. Over time, the range of phenomena that various groups of behavior therapists have been willing to consider as important has changed and broadened, producing a number of different schools within the behavioral movement. At present, there are five different schools (Redd et al. 1979), distinguishable in large measure on the basis of their views of cognition.

The first group, the applied behavior analysts, is the one most closely associated with Skinner's (1938) radical behaviorism. This position holds that only environmental and individual phenomena which are *observable* are meaningful objects of study. While behavior may be studied, because it may be seen, "private events" such as cognitions and emotions are regarded as being epiphenomenal, never a cause or mediator of behavior, and consequently irrelevant to the treatment of human functioning. Applied behavior analysis is best described as a systematic methodology for the investigation of overt behavior, whereby one systematically alters selected aspects of the environment and carefully observes the behavior of persons in that environment to identify environment-behavior functional relationships. Applied behavior analysis has been called naive for excluding all cognitive processes from consideration. Nevertheless, it has proven itself to be impressively powerful in application, as a tool of both assessment and therapy (See Kazdin 1980).

Learning, or conditioning, theory is the second major school. It is most closely associated with the clinical work of Joseph Wolpe (Wolpe and Lazarus 1966) and regards behavior problems as the result of one of two forms of learning: classical conditioning or operant conditioning. Classical conditioning is the name of the process by which an originally neutral stimulus in the environment comes to elicit a certain reaction after being repeatedly paired with a second stimulus that reflexively elicits a reaction closely related to the conditioned one. Operant conditioning is the name of the process by which the rate of a certain behavior is altered by controlling the consequence that follows its occurrence. Therapies from the learning, or conditioning theory school use these two forms of learning to replace problematic behaviors with adaptive ones.

The learning theory approach differs from applied behavior analysis in that it does make great use of one unobservable state—anxiety—in its explanations for behavior. However, the schools are similar in their views that the external, observable environment is the ultimate cause of behavioral events and that thoughts, or cognitions, are unimportant.

Social learning theory is the third major school of behavioral thought and is best reflected in the work of Bandura (1969). This school agrees that the processes described by classical and operant conditioning are important but argues that a third, and more powerful, process is important as well.

This third process is known as cognitive mediation, and it involves the symbolic coding of environment-organism interactions, the cognitive testing of hypotheses about the rules governing behavioral consequences in given situations, and the generation of rules and strategies to govern enacted behavior in specified situations—activities loosely known as thinking. Social learning theory argues that behavior can be changed indirectly by watching the behavior of others with its attendant cues and consequences or, put differently, by altering cognitions alone. The view that learning, and therefore behavior change, can occur by vicarious or symbolic means alone introduces a much wider role for cognitions than is present in the applied behavior analytic or learning theory schools.

The fourth major school of behavioral thought, cognitive behavior therapy (Mahoney 1974; Meichenbaum 1977), gives the widest formal recognition to the role of cognitions in behavior. Cognitive behavior therapists agree with adherents of the other behavioral schools that human behavior is best viewed as occurring in response to the environment; they differ, however, in their view of the environment, which is a difference with major implications for views of other concepts as well. The environment is not considered to be objective; cognitive behavior therapists view behavior as responsive to the environment *as perceived and interpreted by the behavior.* It is important within this view to attend not just to behaviors and environments, but to the attitudes, values, and interests of clients that may influence the meanings their behaviors and environments have for them. The role of cognitions in behavior, then, is extended beyond the point of mediation and in fact cognitions are regarded as true causal elements. Therefore, many therapeutic techniques are directed toward changing how individuals interpret and label their environments rather than properties of the external environment per se. The approach is behavioral in that problematic cognitions which are identified are treated directly rather than regarded as symptomatic of more fundamental problems.

The fifth distinct school among behavior therapists may be called eclectic, or broad-spectrum, behavior therapy (Lazarus 1976). This school is currently the largest of the individual schools (Swan and MacDonald 1978). Its adherents are bound not by an allegiance to any particular theoretical views of certain concepts but by an openness to using any empirically validated technique that fits the needs of an individual case. Eclectic or broad-spectrum behavior therapists draw freely from the methods of the other behavioral schools as well as the more traditional therapies. The approach is a pragmatic one, and the choice of technique is based on the data of each specific case rather than the preexisting theory. Eclectic behavior therapists regularly include the full range of cognitive and affective variables, as well as overt behavior and environmental contingencies, in their case assessments. Because of its willingness to adopt whatever methods are useful, eclectic behavior therapy offers a remarkably flexible approach to a wide range of clinical problems.

BASIC PRINCIPLES COMMON TO THE BEHAVIORAL APPROACH

Throughout the evolution of the various schools of behavior therapy, several basic principles have been conserved. It is this basic core of ideas that binds the schools together into a single therapy movement.

Problematic behavior is held as the focal concern. Behavior therapists reject the notion that problematic behavior has importance only as a symptom of some deeper and more meaningful problem or as a reflection of some fixed path of development gone astray. Behavior research suggests that problematic behavior is learned and maintained by the same principles as is other behavior (Ayllon and Haughton 1968; Ullmann and Krasner 1974) and that more adaptive patterns of behavior can be taught, directly, to supplant it.

As might be guessed, the definition of what constitutes behavior differs across the various behavioral schools. Applied behavior analysts represent the most restrictive approach and admit only overt motoric responses which can be reliably recorded by more than one observer. Cognitive behavior therapists, at the other end of the continuum, include problematic cognitions (thoughts, beliefs, attitudes) under the label of behavior and assess and treat them directly. Whether cognitions are regarded as behavior or not, however, all behavioral approaches are marked by their concern with directly assessing and altering the behavior they have identified as problematic.

The behavioral approaches are also tied by their common use of the functional analysis of behavior (Bijou and Peterson 1968; Kanfer and Soslow 1969) as their primary assessment strategy. This strategy involves first developing a clear definition of the problematic behavior and then identifying the environmental events that regularly precede and follow it. This approach is used because behavior is regarded as functional within its surrounding environment so that behavior change requires knowledge of the function problematic behavior serves. It is a problematic behavior's current function, rather than its apparent symbolism or hypothetical meaning, which gives the critical information about how it can be altered.

Regardless of school, behavior therapists are committed to the empirical validation of treatments, both as they are applied clinically and as they are developed experimentally. Whenever possible, assessments are conducted throughout treatment so that levels of the problematic behavior will be conspicuous to therapist and client alike, infusing accountability. Failures to find change are cues to reconstruct the therapy program, and knowledge of the degree of change allows continuous tailoring of treatments to match the client's status over the course of therapy.

BEHAVIOR THERAPY WITH THE AGING

Cautions in Using the Behavioral Approach with the Aging

The third unifying theme mentioned above, namely, maintaining continuous assessment of treatment effects, gives behavior therapy an inherent governor: if the treatment is not working or is somehow making things worse, the therapist and client will quickly know it. Even so, it is of course better to avoid using a nonhelpful procedure in the first place than it is to recognize that a procedure is not working, and therefore, some caution should be exercised before implementing a behavior change program.

First, the persons planning, implementing, and monitoring the treatments should be qualified to do so. Behavior therapy, done correctly, is not a simple approach. If on-site personnel are not trained in behavioral procedures, consultation with other professionals who are so trained should precede any intervention. Second, even trained behavior therapists should not institute behavioral treatments automatically, without evaluation of whether other psychological or medical therapies might be more appropriate. This concern is particularly important in work with the aging, for whom adequate treatments often require a multidisciplinary approach (Kleh, Lange, Karu, and Amos 1978).

Behavior therapy, like any treatment, should not be applied unilaterally. It should be implemented only following consultation with the recipient, or his or her agent, about whether treatment is justified, whether the specific treatment planned is acceptable, and whether the treatment goals are perceived as beneficial to the person receiving treatment (Kazdin 1980). While behavioral technology may be used to render people easier to manage, as are medical and physical technologies (Covert, Rodrigues, and Solomon 1977), such actions cannot be construed as therapeutic; they are no more a part of behavior therapy than forced sterilization is of medicine (MacDonald 1977).

Behavior Therapy with Aging Outpatients

One of the places where behavior therapy may be most useful is in providing outpatient services for aging individuals. As a group, the aging are currently underserved by outpatient mental health services. They comprise roughly 10% of the nation's population, yet account for 2% of the client load in outpatient groups (Kucharski, White, and Schratz 1979). Part of the reason for this may be found in the aging's documented reluctance to begin using any new services which community mental health centers, for instance, would be, even when these services are free (Barney and Neukom 1979). But the primary reason for the aging's under-representation is very probably the professional's active avoidance of treating (Garfinkel 1975) or reluctance to treat (MacDonald 1973) the mental health problems of the aging. The reason for this reluctance cannot be found in the nature of the problems aging persons present, for older persons have been found to be significantly less likely than are younger ones to be referred for psychological help even given the same behavioral and physical problems (Kucharski, White, and Schratz 1979). While some of the reason would certainly be age prejudice, currently known as ageism (Kalish 1979), at least some of the reason would also doubtlessly be the inapplicability of therapeutic approaches requiring long-term treatment and historical integrations with this group—approaches which, until recently, have constituted the only treatment alternative.

Many features of behavior therapy, including its focus on the present, make it uniquely appropriate for working with outpatient clients:

> Psychotherapy with the aged should not involve the task of reconstructing the patient's basic personality. Rather, the purpose of intervention in the majority of cases is to help the patient cope with problems (Brink 1977, p. 274).

Pfeiffer (1979) provides a detailed description of how the therapy should begin. As with any age group, establishing rapport is a critical prerequisite to extracting useful information during assessment as well as instituting effective interventions during treatment:

> The initial message to be communicated to the distressed elderly patient should be warmth, interest, and concern..., an open smile, a welcoming outreaching gesture, some physical contact. (Pfeiffer 1979, p. 25).

After establishing rapport, the starting point is learning what has brought the person to therapy. If there is strong evidence that the distress is of recent onset and is a response to specific, identifiable circumstances, a package known as *crisis intervention* (Rappaport 1977) is particularly appropriate. The principle elements of this approach include: (1) providing a nonjudgmental but controlled opportunity to ventilate affect; (2) effectively communicating correct empathic understanding of the experience and its associated feelings; (3) exploring the likely outcomes of alternative courses of action; (4) selecting one course of action and planning its execution in detail, and; (5) setting an occasion to collaboratively evaluate the effects of the executed option and, if they were not entirely remedial, to establish an additonal plan of action.

Brink (1977) reports a case illustrating this approach:

> A 64 year old widow complained that she lacked the desire to go on living. She said she spent most of the day sitting idly or taking naps. She

had the habit of waking up in the middle of the night and contemplating the most effective means of suicide (Brink 1977, p. 273).

The problematic behavior in this case was an affect, depression, which is thought to be one of the more common problems for this age group (Poliquin and Staker 1977). Inquiry about onset and the circumstances surrounding it indicated that it was apparently precipitated by a change in the woman's life style, namely a gradual decrease in the amount of time she spent in enjoyable activities. Brink (1977), agreeing with behavioral formulations of depression (Craighead 1979; Lewisohn, 1974), notes that "treatment for depression should be primarily supportive and should encourage the person's activity" (p. 275). This formulation regards depression as resulting from a deficiency in enjoyable activities, a deficiency which is self-perpetuating in that once a person becomes unhappy, it is difficult for them to initiate activities which would literally make them feel better and therefore, eliminate the depression. Treatment involves providing structures to make increased activity more likely (since depressed persons will generally not increase their activity levels spontaneously), and doing so supportively (since depressed individuals are likely to be experiencing distorted, negative thoughts about themselves) (Beck 1976).

In the case described by Brink (1977), treatment involved identifying activities which might be pleasurable both inherently and because of their exposure to opportunities for socially interacting with others:

> From the very first session, a major effort was made to assess and improve her activity. She was encouraged to increase her visits to her friends..., perform daily physical exercises, take an interest in gardening, and participate in more religious activities (p. 275-276).

She was asked to keep a record of her daily activities, for several reasons. First, the record provided an assessment of whether treatment was working, a record which was visible to both her therapist and herself. Second, her record served to remind her of her task and her success at it. And finally, when shared with the therapist, her record allowed for the therapist's giving of support as a reward for her efforts. The treatment was effective. Brink (1977) reports that the depression lifted within a matter of several weeks and did not recur.

Like depression, senility is a problem often associated with the aging. And like depression, senility may often have its source in reversible environmental circumstances. The fact that senility is not always irreversible, and is not always a function of cortical deterioration, is less well known than it should be. Unfortunately, certain problematic behaviors such as wandering, confusion, or marked mood changes are often translated into diagnoses of senility simply because of the person's age, without further examination of his or her psychobiological problems. Kleh, Lange, Karu, and Amos (1978) report a case illustrating this point, as well as the near tragic consequences such misdiagnoses can have:

> A retired woman was about to be sent to a nursing home after exhibiting all the overt symptoms of senility; she was agitated, had a short attention span, and behaved in strange ways. She even shared her thoughts with an imaginary roommate. In reality, however, she was suffering from an agitated depression, resulting in large part from her isolation from her daughter, who was unable to take care of her at home. Yet, for many weeks, the real nature of the problem was not detected, and the label of senility appeared to be appropriate (p. 735).

In this situation, a functional analysis of behavior was sufficient to establish that the problematic behaviors, when evaluated in context, were a result of environmental conditions and were treatable with behavior therapy techniques. This is not an uncommon circumstance (Yesavage 1979).

There are also situations, however, where senile-like behaviors are treatable, but where neither the cause nor the cure is psychological. These situations include occasions when the problem is resulting from one of several possible medical sources including drug toxicity (which is ironically most likely to result with the drugs the aging are most likely to have prescribed), metabolic and endocrine disorders, nutritional disorders, and systemic infections (Yesavage 1979).

Since instances of senile-like behaviors resulting from treatable organic problems are not uncommon (Ounn 1977), it is essential to have these alternative causes considered by someone competent to evaluate them. A case illustrating the importance of securing a medical consultation prior to instituting a psychological therapy for a potentially medical problem was reported by Kleh and his associates (1978).

> In one case, an apparently psychotic 69-year-old man had gained 60 pounds, started to put garbage in the refrigerator, and became disoriented in all spheres. A multidisciplinary team made a thorough evaluation of the patient and identified a severe medical problem—congestive heart failure. When both medical and psychiatric symptoms were taken into consideration, the team determined the man was suffering from acute organic brain syndrome secondary to congestive heart failure. When his heart condition was treated, his weight decreased significantly, and his confusion cleared (p. 736).

While depression and senile-like symptoms are two problems thought to be particularly common with the aging (Poliquin and Straker 1977), it is important to remain sensitive to the fact that other problems troubling younger persons touch this age group as well. Behavioral treatments, which are determined primarily by the problem requiring treatment and the circumstances surrounding its occurrence rather than demographic characteristics of the person presenting it, have been developed for a wide variety of clinical circumstances. They are as applicable with an older person as they are with a younger one. A case reported by Garfinkel (1979) illustrates this point.

A seventy-five year old woman presented to Garfinkel (1979) with persistent feelings of tightness in the chest, choking, and a lack of breath. Questions designed to allow a functional analysis of the problematic behaviors indicated that they generally occurred together and whenever the woman had to "act on her own," especially with strangers. The problems were conceptualized as facets of an anxiety reaction; they were treated using systematic desensitization, a standard behavioral treatment for anxiety experienced in response to clearly specifiable stimuli. The treatment, which extended over several months, was completely successful.

Although behavioral treatments have been effective with problems presented by aging outpatients, as they have been with problems presented by younger ones, it is perhaps every helping professional's dream that outpatient treatment would become unnecessary by virtue of problems being prevented before they occur. The notion of prevention, popularized with the increase in interest in community mental health more than a decade ago (Nietzel, Winett, MacDonald, and Davidson, 1977), was adopted from public health concepts which argued that the most effective treatment for problems such as smallpox was prevention before the fact (Rappaport 1977).

A SURVEY OF THE PREVENTATIVE APPROACH

The preventative or community mental health approach is particularly compatible with behavior therapy, since one of the major principles of this approach is that problems are influenced by environmental factors, factors that can be altered before the problem erupts. One model which may prove particularly useful in this effort, although still a very new one, is the stress adaptation model (Palmore, Cleveland, Nowlin, Ramm, and Siegler 1979). This model asserts that problems result from an interaction between environmental disruptions and environmental supports. Stated differently, problems result from disruptions in one's living situation which are not buffered by environmental resources available concurrently. The implication is that problems may be prevented by developing environmental supports which will minimize the negative impact of foreseeable potential disruptions.

Palmore, Cleveland, Nowlen, Ramm, and Siegler (1979) report data suggesting the utility of this model. For aging males, retirement is ordinarily followed by more negative changes than any other life event: it is followed by decreases in life satisfaction, increases in psychosomatic symptoms, and decreases in feelings of usefulness and self-esteem. However, neither retirement nor either of the other two less severe but still serious common disruptions for aging persons, health crises and social crises, have been found to result in long term negative effects *if* the persons experiencing them had social environments which included medical and social resources (Palmore et al. 1979; see also Conner, Powers, and Bultena 1979; Laing, Kahanz, and Doherty 1980; Linn and Hunter 1979; Markides and Martin 1979). It is possible then, to prevent negative results from events that cannot themselves be prevented; the solution is found in the provision of compensatory supports.

Prevention with the aging is a very new concept, and treatments directed toward this end have not been evaluated carefully (See Liviton and Santa 1979). One program has appeared in the literature, however, which looks especially promising. Ruffini and Todd (1979) established a program whose overriding goal was to precipitate the development of a peer support network among the aging. Their concrete goals were threefold: (1) providing information and referral services through a newsletter, monthly meetings with guest speakers, and periodic telephone contacts; (2) encouraging increased levels of social interactions among the elderly; and (3) encouraging self-peer help among members of the group. These concrete goals were accomplished—but not by Ruffini and Todd (1979). Elderly volunteers, recruited by Ruffini and Todd, independently canvassed their neighborhoods to compile lists of every person over the age of sixty and then assumed the responsibility for hand delivering monthly newsletters to them.

Unfortunately, no formal evaluation of the Ruffini and Todd (1979) program was reported. As developed, however, the program was somewhat self-correcting, in that it was directed by the aging themselves and evolved in response to the circumstances that it found within this population (Ward 1979). In fact, the program's strength, above all else, lay in its nature of responding to the stated needs of the population and consequently avoiding a problem that Kalish (1979) has termed the new form of ageism:

> The message of the New Age-ism seems to be that ''we'' understand how badly you are being treated, that ''we'' have the tools to improve your treatment, and that if you adhere to our program, ''we'' will make your life considerably better (Kalish 1979, p. 398).

As Kalish (1979) observes, this sort of new-agist communication, which is regretably becoming more common, transmits a lack of equality, and a lack of faith in the listener's ability to manage her or his own affairs. While intended to be beneficial, it runs the risk of seeing and perhaps creating need where there is none.

As long as the individual's right to refuse treatment, particularly preventive treatment, is preserved, the concept of prevention for recipients who would like it is extremely appealing on humanitarian grounds. Like other models of service delivery, however, it would involve considerable expense to establish and maintain. Although there are some indications that a preventive model might be more cost effective than a remedial one once it was established (Mims, Thomas, and Conroy 1977), the start-up costs would be greater (see Skelton 1977). As Burkhardt (1977) has noted, unfortunately the best service systems are also often the most expensive ones, and it remains a political decision as to whether the societal gains outweigh the societal costs.

BEHAVIOR THERAPY WITH THE INSTITUTIONALIZED AGING

Of the twenty-three million aging people currently living in the United States, (Kalish 1979), only 5% live in institutions or group quarters (Mindel 1979). However, estimates indicate that nearly 40% of the current adult population will be institutionalized in a nursing home at some point during the last ten years of their lives (Reed and Glamser 1979), 15% for a period longer than six months. The largeness of these latter two statistics may seem surprising; their size results from the fact that nursing homes are often the only treatment alternative for aging persons who need any sort of assistance (Bayne and Caygill 1977; MacDonald 1973; Redick 1974; Schmidt, Reinhardt, Kane, and Olson 1977). Furthermore, the size of these statistics may very well not decrease in the coming years, even if preventative models become well developed and if noninstitutional geriatric treatment centers become more common (see Mitchell 1978; Weissert 1978), because the number of persons over eighty who typically need extensive care, is projected to double in the next two decades (Glick 1979). Pinker (1980) has not been alone in noting that, like it or not, institutional treatment for the aging will remain necessary for some time to come.

As early as 1966 (Cautela 1966; Kastenbaurm 1968), empirically oriented clinical psycholgists were suggesting the potential utility of behavior therapy for treating the institutionalized aging. Although the area has been explored less frequently than would be desirable, a number of studies show that behavior therapy is, in fact, effective in this context. Aging institution-wide or ward-wide programs have focused on three major areas: exercise, meaningful activity, and social interaction. A variety of behavior problems have been treated with individualized programs.

Increasing levels of physical exercise has been an especially popular focus of study as well as a worthwhile one, since the usual sedentary life observed in total-care institutions produces muscular atrophy and general physical deterioration (Comstock, Meyers, and Folsom 1969; Quilitch 1974). Various investigators (Adams and deVries 1973; DeCarlo 1977; Elsayad, Ismail, and Young 1980; Libb and Clements 1969; Sandel 1978) have instituted behavioral programs which provide structures and/or rewards to increase physical exercise and to effect increases in levels of physical activity. Among the benefits noted have been increased cognitive ability (Elsayad et al. 1980; Powell 1974), improved general health (DeCarlo et al 1977), and increased levels of social interaction (Sandel 1978).

Increasing levels of meaningful activity has been a second focus. Mc-Clannahan and Risley (1973; 1974), Quilitch (1975), and Quattrochi-Tobin and Jason (1980) demonstrated that activity levels could be increased significantly by structuring the environment so that environmental opportunities were available. MacDonald and Settin (1978) found that structuring opportunities for meaningful activity increased activity levels, levels of life satisfaction, and levels of social involvement. MacDonald, Davidowitz, Gimbel, and Foley (1978) demonstrated also that using staff attention to reinforce participation in activities increased activity levels over those observed when opportunities to be active were provided without staff attention.

Social interaction has been the target of a final set of group investigations. Hoyer, Kafer, Simpson, and Hoyer (1974), Mueller and Atlas (1972), and MacDonald (1978) have independently demonstrated that levels of social interaction can be increased by giving participants rewards for interacting. Brickel (1979) reported that simply providing a "conversation piece," which in this case was a pet cat, could both increase levels of social interaction and ward activity. Sommer and Ross (1958) found that rearranging the lobby furniture so that chairs were near and facing one another more than doubled the rate of between resident conversation.

CONCLUSION

We have tried to introduce the reader to some of the potential uses of behavior therapy with the aging. Behavior therapy offers an extremely flexible approach to the problems of this, or any, population. It contains an assessment technique which is especially helpful in discriminating psychological from physiological problems, and which lends itself directly to the formulation and revision of individualized treatment programs. It offers a number of treatment options which, while no match for the complexity and range of human behavior, at least better approximates them than any of the monolithic therapy approaches. Finally, it is amenable for use on any of several levels (outpatient, prevention, and inpatient) and thus, can be tailored to the client rather than requiring clients to be tailored to it.

Behavior therapy also offers several pragmatic advantages in an increasingly cost conscious world. It is amenable for use by *supervised* paraprofessionals, thus reducing unit costs and appropriately expanding the availability of treatment services. It also embodies a way to minimize the new ageism in that it would be quite appropriate and possible for the elderly to absorb behavioral technologies into their own expertise and therefore, establish and maintain their own programs.

Whether behavior therapy *should* be used as a treatment approach for the aging has been, and continues to be, the focus of much theoretical speculation (see MacDonald 1977). The body of empirical demonstrations and evaluations of the usefulness of behavior therapy with the aging is increasing rapidly, however, and the evidence clearly suggests that behavior therapy is a useful, even powerful, approach to the problems of aging citizens. While many older Americans live out their lives in a reasonably full and happy manner, the life circumstances of some are less than optimal. The chronic lack of financial resources, increasing physical limitations, and erosion of social role and control for these persons all work together to produce a significant amount of life stress, a stress which is all the harder to handle well if the elderly are unable to obtain help from appropriate psychotherapeutic sources. Behavior therapy offers a flexible approach to many of these problems; given its effectiveness, and the cost of leaving these problems untreated, it seems most reasonable to employ behavior therapy as a treatment alternative whenever appropriate.

References

Adams, G. M., & deVries, H. A. Physiological effects of an exercise training regimen upon women aged 52 to 79. *Journal of Gerontology,* 1973, *28:* 50-55.

Ayllon, T., & Haughton, E. Modification of symptomatic verbal behavior of mental patients. *Behavior Research and Therapy,* 1964, *2:* 87-97.

Bandura, A. *Principles of behavior modification.* New York: Holt, Rinehart, & Winston, 1969.

Barney, J. L. & Neukom, I. E. Use of arthritis care by the elderly. *Gerontologist,* 1979, *19:* 548-554.

Bayne, J. R. D., & Caygill, J. Identifying needs and services for the aged. *Journal of the American Geriatrics Society,* 1977, *25:* 264-268.

Beck, A. T. *Cognitive therapy and the emotional disorders.* New York: International Universities Press, 1976.

Bijou, S. W., & Peterson, R. F. The psychological assessment of children: A functional analysis. In P. McReynolds (ed.), *Advances in psychological assessment.* Vol. 2, New York: Science and Behavior Books, 1972.

Brickel, C. M. The therapeutic roles of cat mascots with a hospital-based geriatric population. *Gerontologist,* 1979, *19:* 368-372.

Brink, T. L. Brief psychotherapy: A case report illustrating its potential effectiveness. *Journal of the American Geriatrics Society,* 1977, *25:* 273-276.

Burkhardt, J. E. Evaluating information and referral services. *Gerontologist,* 1979, *19:* 28-33.

Cautela, J. R. Behavior therapy and geriatrics. *Journal of Genetic Psychology,* 1966, *108:* 9-17.

Comstock, R. L., Meyers, R. L. & Folsom, J. C. Simple physical activities for the elderly. *Hospital Community Psychiatry,* 1969, *20:* 377-389.

Conner, K. A., Powers, E. A., & Bultena, G. L. Social interaction and life satisfaction: an empirical assessment of late-life patterns. *Journal of Gerontology,* 1979, *34:* 116-121.

Covert, A. B., Rodrigues, T., & Solomon, K. The use of mechanical and chemical restraints in nursing homes. *Journal of the American Geriatrics Society,* 1977, *25:* 85-89.

Craighead, W. E. Away from a unitary model of depression. *Behavior Therapy,* 1980, *11:* 122-128.

DeCarlo, T. J., Castiglione, L. V., & Cavusoglu, M. A program of balanced physical fitness in the preventive care of elderly ambulatory patients. *Journal of the American Geriatrics Society,* 1977, *25:* 331-334.

Elsayad, M., Ismail, A. H., & Young, R. J. Intellectual differences of adult men related to age and physical fitness before and after an exercise program. *Journal of Gerontology,* 1980, *35:* 383-387.

Garfinkel, R. The reluctant therapist. *Gerontologist,* 1975, *15:* 138-141.

Garfinkel, R. Brief behavior therapy with an elderly patient. *Journal of Geriatric Psychiatry,* 1979, *12:* 101-109.

Glick, P. C. The future marital status and living arrangements of the elderly. *Gerontologist,* 1979, *19:* 301-309.

Gunn, A. E. Mental impairment in the elderly: Medical-legal assessment. Journal of the American Geriatrics Society, 1977, *25:* 193-198.

Hoyer, W. J., Kafer, R. A., Simpson, S. C., & Hoyer, F. W. Reinstatement of verbal behavior in elderly mental patients using operant procedures. *Gerontologist,* 1974, *14:* 149-152.

Kalish, R. A. The new ageism and the future models: A polemic. *Gerontologist,* 1979, *19:* 398-402.

Kanfer, F. H., & Saslow, G. Behavioral diagnosis. In C. M. Franks (ed.), *Behavior therapy: appraisal and status,* New York: McGraw-Hill, 1969.

Kastenbaum, R. Perspective on the development and modification of behavior in the aged: A developmental-field perspective. *Gerontologist,* 1969, *8:* 280-283.

Kazdin, A. E. Acceptability of time out from reinforcement procedures for disruptive child behavior. *Behavior Therapy,* 1980, *11:* 329-344.

Kleh, J., Lange, P., Karu, E., & Amos, C. Differential diagnosis of the disturbed elderly patient. *Hospital & Community Psychiatry,* 1978: *29,* 735-737.

Kucharski, L. T., White, R. M., Jr., & Schratz, M. Age bias referral for psychological assistance, and the private physician. *Journal of Gerontology,* 1979, *34:* 423-428.

Laing, J., Kahana, E., & Doherty, E. Financial well-being among the aged: A further elaboration. *Journal of Gerontology,* 1980, *35:* 409-420.

Lazarus, A. A. *Multimodal behavior therapy.* New York: Springer, 1976.

Leviton, D. & Santa Maria, L. The adults health and development program: Descriptive and evaluative data. *Gerontologist,* 1979, *19:* 534-543.

Lewinsohn, P. M. A behavioral approach to depression. In R. J. Friedman & M. M. Katz (eds.), *The psychology of depression—contemporary theory and research.* New York: Wiley, 1974.

Libb, J. W., & Clements, C. B. Token reinforcement in an exercise program for hospitalized geriatric patients. *Perceptual and Motor Skills,* 1969, *28:* 957-958.

Linn, M. W., & Hunter, K. Perception of age in the elderly. *Journal of Gerontology,* 1979, *34:* 46-52.

MacDonald, M. L. The forgotton Americans: A sociopsychological analysis of aging and nursing homes. *American Journal of Community Psychology,* 1973, *1:* 272-294.

MacDonald, M. L. The ethics of using behavior modification with the institution-alized aging: a practical analysis. *Journal of Long-Term Care Administration,* 1976, *4:* 42-46.

MacDonald, M. L., Davidowitz, J., Gimbel, B., & Foley, L. M. Environmental programming for the institutionalized aging. Paper presented at the annual meeting of the Association for Advancement of Behavior Therapy, New York, December, 1978.

MacDonald, M. L., & Settin, J. M. Reality orientation versus sheltered workshops as treatment for the institutionalized aging. *Journal of Gerontology,* 1978, *33:* 416-421.

McClannahan, L. E., & Risley, T. R. A store for nursing home residents. *Nursing Homes,* 1973, *22:* 10-11.

McClannahan, L. E., & Risley, T. R. Activities and materials for severely disabled geriatric patients. *Nursing Homes,* 1974, *23:* 19-23.

Mahoney, M. J. *Cognition and behavior modification.* Cambridge, Massachusetts: Ballinger, 1974.

Markides, K. S., & Martin, H. W. A causal model of life satisfaction among the elderly. *Journal of Gerontology,* 1979, *34:* 86-93.

Meichenbaum, D. *Cognitive-behavior modification.* New York: Plenum, 1977.

Mims, R. B., Thomas, L. L. & Conroy, M. V. Physician house calls: a comple-ment to hospital-based medical care. *Journal of the American Geriatrics Society,* 1977, *25:* 28-34.

Mindel, C. H. Multigenerational family households: Recent trends and implica-tions for the future. *Gerontologist,* 1979, *19:* 456-463.

Mitchell, J. B. Patient outcomes in alternative long care settings. *Medical Care,* 1978 *16:* 439-452.

Mueller, D. J., & Atlas, L. Resocialization of regressed elderly residents: A be-havioral management approach. *Journal of Gerontology,* 1972, *27:* 390-392.

Nietzel, M. J., Winett, R. A., MacDonald, M. L., & Davidson, W. S. *Behavioral approaches to community psychology.* New York: Pergamon, 1977.

Palmore, E., Cleveland, W., Nowlin, J., Ramm, D., & Siegler, I. Stress and adaptation in later life. *Journal of Gerontology,* 1979, *34:* 841-851.

Pfeiffer, E. Handling the distressed older patient. *Geriatrics,* 1979, *34:* 24-32.

Pinker, R. A. Facing up to the eighties: Health & welfare needs of British elderly. *Gerontologist,* 1980, *20'* 273-283.

Poliquin, N., & Straker, M. A clinical psychogeriatric unit: Organization and function. *Journal of the American Geriatrics Society,* 1977, *25:* 135-137.

Powell, R. R. Psychological effects of exercise therapy upon institutionalized geriatric mental patients. *Journal of Gerontology,* 1974, *29:* 157-161.

Quattrochi-Tubin, S., & Jason, L. A. Enhancing social interactions and activity among the elderly through stimulus control. *Journal of Applied Behavior Analysis,* 1980, *13:* 159-163.

Quilitch. H. R. Purposeful activity increased on a geriatric ward through programmed recreation. *Journal of the American Geriatrics Society, 1974, 22:* 226-229.

Quilitch, H. R. A comparison of three staff-management procedures. *Journal of Applied Behavior Analysis,* 1975, *8:* 59-66.

Rappaport, J. *Toward a community psychology: the search for new paradigms.* New York: Holt, Rinehart, & Winston, 1977.

Redd, W. H., Porterfield, A. L., & Anderson, B. L. *Behavior modification,* New York: Random House, 1979.

Redick, R. W. *Patterns of use of nursing homes by the aged mentally ill.* Statistical note 107, NIMH, Rockville, MD, 1974.

Reed, M. B., & Glamser, F. D. Aging in a total institution: The case of older prisoners. *Gerontologist,* 1979, *19:* 354-360.

Ruffini, J. L., Todd, H. F., Jr. A network model for leadership development among the elderly. *Gerontology,* 1979, *19:* 158-162.

Sandel, S. L. Movement therapy with geriatric patients in a convalescent home. *Hospital Community Psychiatry,* 1978. *29:* 730-741.

Schmidt, L. J., Reinhardt, A. M., Kane, R. L., & Olsen, D. M. The mentally ill in nursing homes. *Archives of General Psychiatry,* 1977, *34:* 687-696.

Skelton, D. The future of health care for the elderly. *Journal of the American Geriatrics Society, 1977, 25:* 39-46.

Skinner, B. F. *Behavior of organism,* New York: Appleton-Century-Crofts, 1938.

Sommer, R., & Ross, H. Social interaction on a geriatric ward. *International Journal of Social Psychology,* 1958, *3:* 128-133.

Swan, G. E., MacDonald, M. L. Behavior therapy in practice: A national survey of behavior therapists. *Behavior Therapy,* 1978, *9:* 799-807.

Ullman, L. P. Behavior therapy as social movement. In C. M. Franks (ed.), *Behavior therapy: appraisal and status.* New York: McGraw-Hill, 1969.

Ullmann, L. P., & Krasner, L. *Case studies in behavior modification.* New York: Holt, Rinehart, & Winston, 1965.

Ulmann, L. P., & Krasner, L. *A psychological approach to abnormal behavior,* (2nd ed.). Cliffs, New Jersey: Prentice-Hall, 1975.

Ward, R. A. The meaning of voluntary association participation for older people. *Journal of Gerontology,* 1979, *34:* 438-445.

Weissert, W. G. Costs of adult day care: a comparison to nursing homes. *Inquiry,* 1978, *15:* 10-19.

Wilson, G. T., & O'Leary, K. D. *Principles of behavior therapy.* Englewood Cliffs, New Jersey: Prentice Hall, 1980.

Wolpe, J. & Lazarus, A. A. *Behavior therapy techniques: a guide to the treatment of neurosis.* London: Pergamon Press, 1966.

Yesavage, J. Dementia: Differential diagnosis and treatment. *Geriatrics,* 1979, *34:* 51-62.

8
Therapeutic Design for the Aging

Scott Danford

Therapeutic intervention with the aging can be based upon any one of several models (Canter 1979): including the custodial model which says "let us take care of you;" the prosthetic model which says "let us compensate for your deficiencies"; or the normalization model which says "let us help you achieve your potential." Therapeutic design operates from a model which in many ways represents a synthesis of certain elements from all the others—the habitability model.

For most people the term *habitability* conjures up images of specific design characteristics which insure negotiability for particular user populations—access ramps to entrances for the wheelchair-bound; brail signage systems for the blind; non-slip floor surfaces for the aging. And yet, although these are design features which may contribute to habitability, habitability involves a great deal more than negotiability.

Although concerned with physical design characteristics, the habitability model addresses itself as much to relationships as hardware. It says "let us establish and maintain specific, preferred relationships between the various contributing elements in a situation." Toward this end, certain physical design features may be employed—but as elements of, and not the whole designed solution. For design is more than architecture: it is purposeful intervention; it is knowledge-based intervention for the purpose of establishing and maintaining a preferred situation (Danford 1978a). With most human situations being the product of multiple, interdependent arenas of influence, the idea of establishing and maintaining preferred relationships between people, their behaviors, and their environments through manipulation of physical design elements alone has been generally abandoned. Consequently habitability based therapeutic design extends its interventions to arenas of influence in addition to the architectural environmental. And yet, to engage in habitable, therapeutic design—or knowledge-based intervention for the purpose of establishing and maintaining specific, preferred relationships between these arenas of influence—a rather detailed theoretical understanding of those arenas and their several interrelationships is required.

PERSON-BEHAVIOR-ENVIRONMENT RELATIONS

As with the more traditionally conceived therapeutic interventions, therapeutic design too rests on theoretical underpinnings which influence the what/why/how of designed, therapeutic intervention—particularly with the aging. Being a relatively new, multidisciplinary, intervention oriented field (see figure 1), therapeutic design has generally called upon that segment of its membership from the social and behavioral sciences—par-

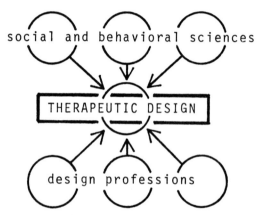

Figure 1.   Therapeutic design as a multi-disciplinary,   intervention-oriented field

ticularly psychology—to provide that theoretical base. Unfortunately, the theories so borrowed have been largely ill-equipped to deal with the subtle, ecological complexities involved in the design of habitable person-behavior-environment relationships: they have generally ignored the physical environment; they have tended to focus exclusively on the individual; and they have often assumed extreme, mutually exclusive positions on the behavior versus cognition and reductionist versus holistic arguments—to name but a few of the problems. Faced with such an array of theories, each with its own unique perspective on—or as some might argue, distortion of—reality, therapeutic design has begun to synthesize the necessary model of the person-behavior-environment relationships by piecing together elements of truth from what might appear to be incompatible theories (see figure 2).

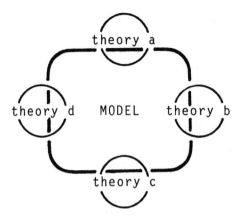

Figure 2.   Piecing together elements of truth to synthesize a model of person-behavior-environment relations

Behavior—Environment

First, it is widely accepted that there is a relatively stable, enduring relationship between behavior and environment (Proshansky et al. 1970). Although few today would embrace a strict architectural/environmental determinism (Mayer 1967; Lang et al. 1974) that is not to say that there is no influence of environment on behavior. Roger Barker (1963a, b) has demonstrated that one of the best pieces of information one could have in order to predict the behavior of a person would be that person's environmental context. There is also mounting evidence indicating that under certain circumstances the physical environment alone may even be capable of exerting a therapeutic influence over some problem behaviors (Richer and Nicoll 1971; Ornitz et al. 1970). Furthermore, it is recognized that this linkage between environment and behavior involves a reciprocal relationship in that not only does environment influence behavior, but that environments can be designed to be responsive to behavioral demands as well. Unfortunately, under most circumstances one cannot intervene therapeutically with any certainty of achieving specific, preferred outcomes when the intervention is based upon this reciprocal environment-behavior relationship alone. There are yet additional determinants of the situation and relationships between those determinants to be considered.

Person—Behavior

Traditionally in the social and behavioral sciences one focuses on the person's control or influence over behavior—particularly in the more humanistic schools of thought. And yet, it is widely acknowledged that behavior can exercise a reciprocal influence on the person as well by serving, at a minimum, as a feedback mechanism to the individual. Again, however, predicting specific, preferred outcomes on the basis of interventions into this reciprocal relationship between person and behavior, when used alone, has a somewhat less than spectacular record of success. This relationship too represents but one of multiple determinants of the situation being considered.

Person—Environment

A third relationship which unquestionably acts as one of the several determinants of any situation is that between person and environment. That the person exerts influence over environment—particularly the designed environment—should come as no surprise as environments today are most often of our own making. What may be less obvious is the reciprocal influence which environment exerts over the person in quite subtle, seemingly imperceptible ways (Maslow and Mintz 1956)—influencing moods, self-concepts, attitudes, values, expectations, perceptions, etc. And yet despite research evidence of this reciprocal relationship, the possibilities of exacting therapeutic interventions based solely on this personal-environment linkage are limited due to the multi-determinant nature of most human situations.

Consequently as reciprocally interdependent determinants of most human situations one finds three primary arenas of influence:

Person—a cognizing organism with values, expectations, capabilities, competencies, attitudes and self-concepts which cannot help but affect the behaviors exhibited as well as the relationships to environment; and organism whose cognitions are undoubtedly influenced by those behaviors and environments in a reciprocal fashion as well;

Environment—a multifaceted package of stimuli (organizational, social, physical, e.g.) which, beyond the reciprocal relationship with the cognitive person, has well established relationships to behavior which probably include both S-R (stimulus-response) and S-O-R (stimulus-organism-response) contingency elements; and

Behavior—an exclusive product of neither the cognitive person nor the contingent environment exclusive, but simultaneous property of both (to some degree) due to the shared reciprocal relationships with each.

Of course, over the years, there have been multiple attempts to combine certain characteristics of these several arenas of influence in an effort to develop an overall model of the person-behavior-environment relationship to be designed. Lewin's (1951) concept of the *life space* in which behavior is seen as a function of the interaction of personality and other individual factors and the perceived environment of the individual combine two unidirectional elements of these relationships. Making those relationships bidirectional to reflect the reciprocal interdependencies involved, and then adding the person-environment reciprocal relationship moves the picture much closer to such contemporary models as Bandura's (1978) person-behavior-environment reciprocal determinism model (see figure 3). Although simple reciprocal determinism does not speak to the dynamic character of the interdependent linkages involved, and therefore remains an oversimplified representation of the relationships, it does provide a basic framework upon which one can expand and to which detail can be added as one considers the possibilities of therapeutic design of these relationships for the aging person.

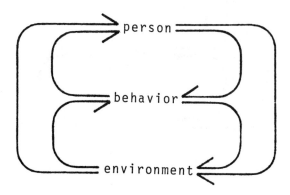

Figure 3.   Bandura's reciprocal determinism model

DYNAMIC RECIPROCAL DETERMINISM

Growing older is popularly linked with a number of negative behavioral characteristics—as if they were an inevitable part of the process of aging. However, the more one understands the complex interdependencies of the situation, the more one is forced to Powell Lawton's (1975, p. 3) conclusion that "relatively few traits typically attributed to the elderly are the inevitable result of chronological aging." In fact often it is found that many of the negative characteristics "are partially or wholly attributable to the... environmental context in which the elderly live." Although such a statement is not necessarily incompatible with the basic reciprocal determinism model of the person-behavior-environment relationships, it does require a detailing of the dynamics involved to explain how environment alone could at anytime exert such an inordinate influence.

People typically think of themselves as exercising direct control over their behaviors. Indeed, much of our society rests on the principal of individual accountability. And yet, the prospect of the aging person—or any person, for that matter—continuously exerting complete, direct, purposeful, conscious control over his/her behaviors during every waking moment of the day is clearly unrealistic. The concentration and stamina required for such a continuous, second by second undertaking would demand superhuman reserves. As an alternative position on the dynamics involved, it counld be suggested that the person actually *monitor* the behavior-environment relationship (see figure 4), adopting a rather passive

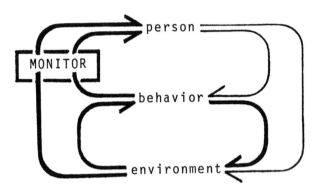

Figure 4.   Monitoring the behavior-environment relationship

stance until such time as s/he chose to reassert control by attempting to *override* the existing behavior-environment relationship (see figure 5).

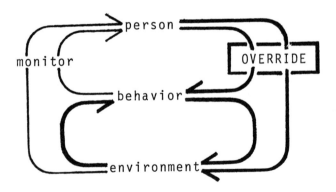

Figure 5.   Overriding the behavior-environment relationship

Typically, one might expect such an attempt at override to occur when the behavior-environment relationship evolves into a pattern substantially at variance with the person's values, expectations and/or capabilities.

The issues of environment challenge and support offer a good example. So long as the amount of challenge or support present in the *demand character*—a combination of constraints, influence and demandingness—of the environment experienced by the aging person is compatible with his/her environmental mastery—a combination of skill, competence, and power/clout—(see figure 6) (e.g., a person of relatively high environmental

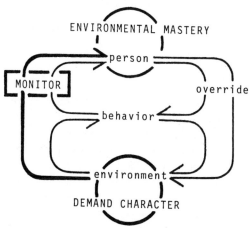

Figure 6.   Monitoring demand character in light of environmental mastery

mastery experiencing an environment whose demand character is higher in challenge and lower in support; a person of relatively low environmental mastery experiencing an environment whose demand character is lower in challenge and higher in support), that person could be expected to monitor the existing behavior-environment relationship and permit it to continue under most circumstances. However, when the amount of challenge or support present in the demand character of the environment experienced by the aging person is incompatible with his/her environmental mastery (e.g., a person of relatively low environmental mastery experiencing an environment whose demand character is higher in challenge and lower in support; a person of relatively high environmental mastery experiencing an environment whose demand character is lower in challenge and higher in support), one might expect this violation of his/her *tolerance threshold,* or willingness/ability to accept deviations from established values, expectations, capabilities, etc., to trigger an attempt to reassert control by *overriding* the existing behavior-environment relationship (see figure 7). Primarily this

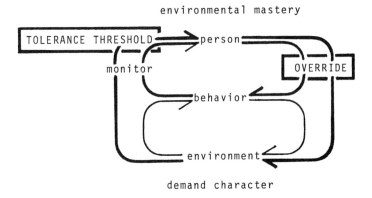

Figure 7.   Violation of tolerance threshold triggering override attempt

would take the form of an attempt to exert direct influence to change either the behavior, the environment, or both. Problems appear when the demand character of the environment perceived to be inappropriate by the aging person is so strong, or the environmental mastery of that person is so weak that the attempt to override becomes a futile exercise. Under these circumstances, the attempt to override will in all likelihood take on the appearance of inappropriate, even maladaptive behavior (see figure 8). For the aging person, such circumstances will typically result in the display of

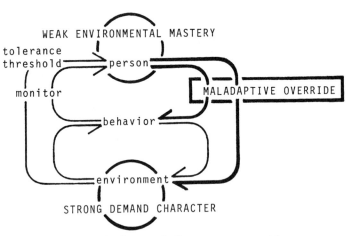

Figure 8.   Maladaptive behavior as a futile attempt at override

negative behavioral characteristics which people too often will write off as intrinsic concommitants of aging. Furthermore, in response to the futility of trying further, the aging person will often simply give up and the override attempts will extinguish. At this point certain others will smile knowingly at this "natural" process of disengagement.

THERAPEUTIC DESIGN

With the basic reciprocal determinism model of the person-behavior-environment relationship now augmented by the addition of a number of concepts required to explain the dynamics involved one who would attempt habitable therapeutic design for the aging at least has a detailed model whose structure and dynamics begin to reflect the several disparate elements of truth which must be acknowledged if specific, preferred outcomes are to be achieved. And the implications for therapeutic design interventions are several.

Given an interdependent, reciprocally-deterministic, multiply-determined, ecological system whose dynamics reflect such considerations as demand character, environmental mastery, tolerance thresholds, monitoring, and override attempts, the prospects for any singular intervention into that situation yielding a singular therapeutic outcome with any predictability becomes remote to say the least. The probability of achieving a specific, preferred person-behavior-environment therapeutic outcome—in the name of habitability or for whatever reason—from a singular intervention into but one of these several arenas of influence is quite limited under most circumstances. To limit oneself to singular interventions into but one arena of influence at any one time—as would be suggested by our hesitancy to violate disciplinary or professional boundaries and identities—would be to kill off any real opportunity to guarantee the design of predictable, therapeutic person-behavior-environment relations. To have any real chance of designing and realizing predictable, habitable person-behavior-environment relationships, one must accept the necessity of multiple, simultaneous, coordinated, design interventions.

Environmental Intervention

The first intervention which comes to many minds is designed environmental intervention (see figure 9). The choice of the term environmental as opposed to architectural is intentional and significant. Although there are numerous architectural design features which can facilitate the establishment of therapeutic person-behavior-environment relationships—particularly for older people (Danford 1978a)—one should resist the temptation to rely overly upon this one arena of influence. Although not discounting its significance, one should remember that the architectural environ-

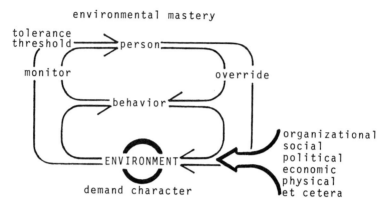

Figure 9.   Environmental intervention

ment is but one of many enviroments with which the aging person must contend. Organizational, social, administrative, and policy concerns all impact upon the aging individual as forms of environment with whose demand character the person must contend. Consequently, a consciously designed policy of coordinated environmental interventions—in additon to the architectural—is mandated to insure internally consistent, or at least compatible, demand character messages from a multi-faceted environment. Mixed demand character messages from uncoordinated environmental factors only present the aging person with a more difficult monitoring task and an increase in the likelihood of threshold tolerance violations with a resultant increase in the probability of inaproppriate,even maladaptive override attempts. Thus it is quite possible to have seemingly good environmental interventions which are undertaken in the name of therapeutic design fall flat or even lead to negative outcomes due to a lack of coordination with other environmental factors which undercut the best efforts.

Person Intervention

A second intervention which is perhaps more often thought of in terms of its therapeutic possibilities is person intervention (see figure 10). Particularly with older people who have been exposed to a lifetime of ageist attitudes, it sometimes becomes necessary virtually to deprogram negative self-concepts and socially suppressed expectations before the potential of designed environmental interventions for creating therapeutic relationships can have any hope of being realized. Without some minimal spark of motivation in the person—a spark which sometimes requires rekindling—those environmental interventions which have been designed to facilitate therapeutic outcomes may never be encountered. Self-doubts and resigna-

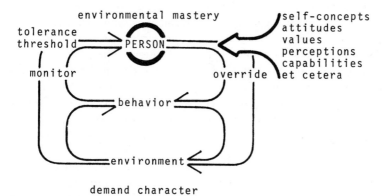

Figure 10.   Person intervention

tion can easily prevent the best designed, therapeutic environmental interventions from ever being experienced.

Behavioral Intervention

Occasionally one may find circumstances such that, despite positive environmental conditions and a willing spirit on the part of the aging person, specific, preferred therapeutic outcomes simply do not occur. In some instances a preferred behavior may have extinguished over time; in other instances a preferred behavior may never have been in the individual's repertoire. These are the conditions under which a third form of intervention may be employed—behavioral intervention (see figure 11). At such times it

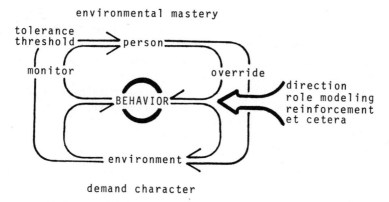

Figure 11.   Behavioral intervention

may be necessary to establish the initial display of a preferred behavior through some combination of direction role modeling, and short-term reinforcement. Although it is often possible to maintain preferred behavior indefinitely with strong enough reinforcement contingencies (i.e., a prosthetic intervention), the therapeutic approach would be to offer only the initial inducements to establish a preferred pattern of behavior and then depend upon the impact of that behavior on the designed person-behavior-environment system to maintain it—assuming, of course, that the pattern of behavior does not significantly violate the aging person's tolerance thresholds with respect to values, expectations, capabilities, etc.

Habitable Outcomes

It is to this last possibility—that the preferred behavioral outcome may in fact be significantly at variance with the individual's values, expectations, capabilities, etc.—that the final implications for therapeutic design intervention speak. There may, on occasion, be a need to require an unpopular behavioral outcome in the establishment or maintenance of habitable person-behavior-environment relationships for the aging person. This is particularly true when powerful, short-term gratification may have to be sacrificed for the long-term good, or when the immediate consequences of the designed relationships are unpleasant—e.g., requiring the mildly arthritic person to ambulate by conventional means for its positive, long-term therapeutic effect despite some temporary discomfort and inconvenience. In such cases, in order to be able to offer some guarantee that the preferred therapeutic outcomes will be realized, a comprehensive, coordinated *management* of the person-behavior-environment relationship (Danford 1978b) is virtually mandated. While maintaining coordinated, therapeutic environmental and behavioral interventions, it may be necessary to prepare the person for the behavior-environment relationship to be experienced by gaining acceptance of that relationship, or at least raising the tolerance threshold for that relationship to lessen the likelihood of futile override attempts. Only through such a holistic management approach which recognizes and is sensitive to the dynamic, ecological interdependencies involved can one hope to control the person-behavior-environment relationship so that therapeutic outcomes are assured. Anything less only provides opportunity for uncontrolled or uncoordinated arenas of influence to frustrate the realization of therapeutic outcomes.

CRITERIA FOR HABITABILITY

After such an extended discussion about the dynamic, reciprocally deterministic nature of the person-behavior-environment relationships and the several types of simultaneous, coordinated interventions required to insure a habitable, therapeutic design one might hope that the criteria for what constitutes such a design would be universally defined. Such is hardly the case. The meaning of habitable, therapeutic intervention is relative to the context in which it is applied. What may prove to be a habitable relationship between person, behavior and environment for one set of circumstances may prove to be quite another for a second. In the same way that the appropriate level of environmental support or challenge must be judged relative to the level of environmental mastery of the person, what constitutes the specific criteria for a particular therapeutic design must be judged relative to the particular person-behavior-environment context with which one is dealing. While no simple listing of universally applicable criteria for what constitutes a habitable, therapeutic outcome can be provided, what can be offered are a few cautions (Williams 1973a) against what might at first glance appear to be ready, sensible criteria.

The first thing to keep in mind is that the therapeutic designer's good intentions by themselves are never enough. Love or good will toward a person offers no guarantee that the designed interventions for that person will yield habitable, therapeutic outcomes. In fact, being a "bleeding heart" for the "poor old people" can very easily be a liability when it comes to making the difficult decisions necessary to insure habitable relationships.

Second, one should be very cautious about accepting some of the more popular criteria which some might suggest for judging the effectiveness of therapeutic designs. In particular, expressions of joy, comfort, satisfaction, pleasure and even happiness may at times prove quite misleading in judging the habitability of designed interventions for the aging person. One must be prepared to accept the fact that wants and needs are not necessarily synonymous when it comes to designing therapeutic relationships for the aging person—or, for that matter, any person.

Third, one must come to recognize that the combined effects of singular therapeutic interventions need not be singular or even additive. Because of the reciprocally interdependent relationships between the several arenas of influence—person, behavior and environment—criteria employed to justify singular interventions into any one arena may not be at all applicable when those interventions are taken in combinations.

And finally, one must be prepared to face unconventional time frames in determining the habitability of a design. With the determination of therapeutic outcomes being such a highly contextual issue, an adequate understanding of the particular person-behavior-environment contextual relationship being addressed is essential. And although one obvious, direct, quantifiable, and objectively verifiable manifestation of those relationships is behavior, it is not just any behavior. Recognizing that discrete, short-term behaviors could reflect only momentary influences from any one of the several arenas of influence, what should be sought are long-term patterns and sequences of behavior which reflect the influences coming from the dynamic interplay of the several arenas of influence—person, environment, and even behavior itself.

THE MATTER OF CONTROL

As should be obvious at this point, therapeutic design for the aging person involves a bit more than simply replacing doorknobs with levers and avoiding blues and greens as orientation colors. Therapeutic design is an intervention-oriented field concerned with establishing and maintaining, even managing, preferred habitable relationships between people, their behaviors and their environments. Toward this end, a considerable degree of control over peoples' lives is necessarily exercised—control which many therapeutic designers have difficulty accepting.

The matter of control is a volatile issue in our society. Somehow control always seems to be popularly associated with oppression, tyranny, and the loss of freedom. Historically that has so often been the case that the popular prejudice against all forms of control, particularly of human behavior, is well ingrained. Regrettable, that puts the therapeutic designer for whom the exercise of control is virtually a tool-in-trade in a somewhat awkward, even sensitive position.

For some designers the preferred response to this situation is not to acknowledge the control which is exercised. They prefer to think of their therapeutic interventions in terms of their *enabling* and *facilitating* roles—as if those were not also forms of control. Still others refer simply to *good* or *user-based* design without reference to the several forms of influence which those designs might yield. Unfortunately, such a refusal to acknowledge the control which is being exercised is actually an exercise in self-delusion. The real danger, of course, is that the designer may actually come to believe this delusion, and as a result fail to recognize the marked impact—positive or negative—which the designed interventions may have on others' lives.

A second response, for those who can/will not delude themselves into denying the existence of the control which they exercise, is to lessen the amount of that control by restricting their therapeutic interventions either to single arenas of influence or to less than completely effective techniques. Somehow it is felt that by denying oneself the option of designing multiple, simultaneous, coordinated interventions, only limited control is being sought due to the acknowledged multideterminant nature of most human situations. Because there are no guarantees that the existing designs of those other arenas of influence will be coordinated or even compatible with the selected therapeutic intervention, and because there are no guarantees that others will select any of the remaining arenas as the target of their limited therapeutic interactions, what this response actually accomplishes is to threaten the therapeutic designer's ability to deliver specific, preferred outcomes with any precision.

The second part of this response, especially for those who cannot deny the imperative to engage in multiple, simultaneous, coordinated interventions, is the tendency to employ something less than the most powerful and effective techniques available. Sensitive to the ever present threat of being indicted as a manipulator of human behavior, these designers are careful not to step over the hypothetical line where the control exercised by the therapeutic interventions would be so all powerful as to strip the aging client of all freedom, autonomy and dignity. Real or not, the person's freedom, autonomy and dignity must somehow be allowed its possible influence over the relationships between person, behavior, and environment, or else the control exercised through the therapeutic interventions supposedly becomes dehumanizing. Whether or not that is the case, what is certain is that willing self-limitation to weaker techniques so that the autonomous person can retain control over the supposed balance of the variance severely threatens the therapeutic designer's ability to deliver those preferred, habitable outcomes with any precison. If control over the person-behavior-environment relationships is to be sought, then it should be attempted with those techniques which can best guarantee success— without regard for the theoretical implications, popular myths, or self-concepts.

A third, somewhat more popular response to this situation is to involve the client in the design decision making process through a participatory approach. By having the aging person contribute to the formulation of specific therapeutic decisions the control exercised by the designs, even if powerful and effective, can still be attributed at least indirectly back to the client. This response requires the therapeutic designer to excercise great care, however. For while there are potential benefits many times associated with participatory approaches to design (e.g., a greater focus on user needs, a lessening of client resistance to change, etc.), an abdication to the client of the therapeutic designer's professional responsibilities can too easily occur. Furthermore, because participatory design does not guarantee user-based design, and because user wants and user needs are not necessarily the same, client participation in the design decision making process can easily threaten the habitability of the therapeutic designs undertaken.

SUMMARY

Therapeutic design for the aging is knowledge-based intervention for the purpose of establishing and maintaining (i.e., controlling) specific, preferred, habitable relationships between aging people, their behaviors, and their environments. Because the relationships between people, behaviors and environments are reciprocally determinant and possess dynamic characteristics enabling any of the three arenas either singly or in combinations to have inordinate influence in certain circumstances, the therapeutic designer is faced with the logical imperative to undertake multiple, simultaneous, coordinated interventions if habitable relationships between the three are to be established and maintained. Toward this end a considerable degree of control over peoples' lives is necessarily exercised—control which therapeutic designers, if they are to function in a professionally responsible fashion, must acknowledge and employ despite the existence of popular sentiment against such action. If control over the person-behavior-environment relationship is to be sought so that habitable therapeutic ends can be achieved, then it should be attempted with those techniques which can best guarantee success. In the business of therapeutic design, anything less only jeopardizes the designer's ability to deliver specific, preferred, habitable outcomes with any precision.

References

Bandura, A. The self system in reciprocal determinism, *American Psychologist,* 1978, 33(4), 344-358

Barker, R. On the nature of the environment. *Journal of Social Issues,* 1963a, *19:* 17-23.

Barker, R. *The stream of behavior.* New York: Appleton, 1963b.

Canter, S. and Canter, D. Building for therapy. In Canter and Canter (eds.) *Designing for therapeutic environments: a review of research.* New York: John Wiley & Sons, 1978.

Danford, S. Designing arenas of influence over elderly behavior. Unpublished paper presented at the 9th Annual Environmental Design Research Association Conference, University of Arizona, Tucson, Arizona, April 1978a.

Danford, S. Designed person-behavior-environment interventions and the elderly: an ecological perspective. Unpublished paper presented at the 57th Annual Meeting of the American Orthopsychiatric Association, Toronto, Ontario, Canada, April 1980.

Danford, S. Managing the person-environment interface. In Weideman and Anderson (eds). *Priorities for environmental design research: part I—selected papers,* pp. 10-13. Washington, D.C.: Environmental Design Research Association, Inc., 1978b.

Lang, J., Burnette, C., Moleski, W., and Vachon, D. Emerging issues in architecture. In J. Lang, et al. (eds), *Designing for human behavior.* Stroudsburg, PA: Dowden, Hutchinson and Ross, Inc., 1974.

Lawton, M. P. An ecological theory of aging, *Journal of Architectural Education,* 1977, *31(1):* 8-10.

Lawton, M. P. *Planning and managing housing for the elderly.* New York: John Wiley & Sons, 1975.

Lewin, K. *Field theory in social science.* New York: Harper and Row, 1951.

Maslow, A., and Mintz, N. Effects of esthetic surroundings. *Journal of Psychology,* 1956, *41:* 247-254.

Mayer, A. *The urgent future.* New York: McGraw-Hill, 1967.

Ornitz, E. et al. Environmental modification of autistic behavior. *Archives of General Psychiatry,* 1970, *22,* 560-565.

Proshansky, H., Ittelson, W., and Rivlin, L. The influence of the physical environment on behavior: some basic assumptions, in H. Proshansky et al. (eds.), *Environmental psychology: man and his physical setting.* New York: Holt, Rinehart and Winston, Inc., 1970.

Richer, R. and Nicholl, S. The physical environment of the mentally handicapped: a playroom for autistic children and its companion therapy project. *British Journal of Mental Subnormality, 1971, 17* (3, part 2): 132-143.

Willems, E. P. Behavioral ecology as a perspective for man-environment research, in W. Preiser (ed.), *Environmental design research, volume two.* Stroudsburg, PA: Dowden, Hutchinson and Ross, Inc., 1973a.

Willems, E. P. Behavior-environment systems: an ecological approach. *Man-Environment Systems, 1973b, 3(2),* 79-110.

Part Three
Discussion

9

Psychotherapy and the Optimizing of Adult Development

James L. Fozard

An applied psychology of aging involves a mix of counseling, therapy, training, and human factors engineering in the framework of a transactional view of changing person-environment relationships in adulthood. Using this concept the role of psychotherapy and counseling is identified in areas of health, work, leisure, memory, and perception.

A useful context for adapting, utilizing, and evaluating psychotherapeutic approaches to the treatment of mental illness in the elderly is the transactional analysis of adult development elaborated in various ways by Lawton and Nahemow (1973), Fozard and Thomas (1973), Riegel (1977), and Baltes and Willis (1977). The transactional view states that in essence person-environment relationships change over adulthood and that the optimal therapeutic approach should consider both environmental and psychological interventions.

Variations in living and working environments—the nature of the neighborhood, the distance between home and work, and perhaps most importantly, the allocation of common space and personal space in homes—differentially affect the styles in which the typical behavior patterns are played out. A developmental view of the interplay between variations in environments and the activities of children and adults who are themselves in different stages of development requires an environment which will optimize the way in which those same people, when older respond to the challenges of retirement, their children's leaving home, and so on.

The possibilities for intervention need not be limited to the perspective of environmental manipulation. Many individual differences in personality, self-expression, and interest patterns observed in old age are predictable from psychological assessments made earlier in the adult life span (cf. Newgarten 1971). An applied psychology of aging should accordingly plan to utilize information about such individual differences which would aid persons in understanding their styles of coping with and adapting to problem situations that arise at different life-course transitions (cf. Schaie and Schaie 1977). Developing an applied psychology involving a balance between environmental intervention and individual counseling for adults represents a significant opportunity for psychologists.

Recent theoretical analysis of aging (Lawton and Nahemow 1973; Fozard and Thomas 1975), under the rubric of an "ecological view of aging," as well as data (Blenker 1967) show that an environment that unduly increases an elderly person's dependence on environmental props and the ministerings of others may well promote irreversible losses of self-sufficiency and independent living.

A developmental analysis of environmental design implies that persons of different ages will not adapt to changes in the environment in the same way. As individuals age, they will be exposed relatively more to certain classes of environments than to others. Accordingly, an elderly person is likely to be better adapted to some situations than to others.

One consequence of being well-adapted to an environment is that a person makes better use of the information it contains in making decisions and in remembering information. Another consequence is that one may experience a substantial disruption in behavior if there is a radical change in that environment. The results of a study by Simon (1964) dramatically illustrate how such a change can differentially affect the behavior of young and old adults. Simon related nurses' ratings of six types of patient activity to age and length of stay in a general, medical, and surgical hospital. Patients were classified into three age groups: 16-53, 54-70, and 71-96; the length of stay in the hospital was divided into thirds. The data indicate that the oldest patients became progressively more idle, isolated, and socially withdrawn with prolonged hospitalization, while the younger and middle-aged patients increased their communications and occupied leisure. The results suggest how a vicious circle might evolve from the elderly's perception of their capabilities and the various "prognoses" given to them by professional staff.

The results of Simon's (1964) study point to the need to redesign the psychosocial environment of general medical hospitals to facilitate the treatment of older persons. Moos and his associates (Moos, Shelton, and Petty 1973; Moos and Houts 1968; Moos and Lemke 1980) describe studies well known to illustrate how differences in the social climate and attitudes fostered in an environment may, in and of themselves, greatly affect the success of a treatment program.

Psychological well-being is the result of an interplay between physical and mental health and the instrumental and expressive aspects of leisure and work. Our desires, fears, and expectations for our own aging are shaped partly by the models of aging provided by elderly parents, relatives, and friends and partly by our own choices of activities over the adult years. One goal of an applied psychology of aging should be to help individuals to recognize the full range of choices of activity that indeed affect the way in which they age. The need to understand age differences in communication (Dowd 1980) is important both for self-understanding and therapeutic skill.

Psychologists concerned with therapy and counseling should base some of their efforts on the problems associated with normal transitions in life. Aging brings with it losses in relatives, resources, and roles as well as some increases in psychological stresses that may accompany those changes. A timely distribution of relatively positive mental health interventions may obviate the need for crisis intervention in later life for many persons.

The degree of choice about one's pattern of aging is increasing continuously because of improvements in health care, industrial technology, flexibility in work schedules, legislation regarding retirement, and advances in our knowledge about adult development. In the following sections the role of psychotherapy and counseling will be related to health, work and leisure, perception, and cognition.

HEALTH

For good reason, the desire for maintenance of good health consistently emerges as the most important item in surveys of the concerns of the elderly. The energy and motivation to identify and initiate new activities during middle and old age is largely determined by physical health.

Present knowledge about the relationship between disease and aging suggests that individuals have a fair degree of control over some factors that increase the likelihood of our reaching an old age—for example, diet, exercise, weight control, styles of reacting to stressful situations, and habits relative to the use of tobacco, alcohol, and drugs.

At present, the possibilities for early medical detection and intervention for many diseases associated with aging are limited (Spark 1976). While the value of some public health interventions is well established, their implementation is not easy. For example, public education efforts relative to choices about the use of tobacco, alcohol, and drugs, and "fast food" have met with limited success. On the positive side, it is evident from the increasing interest in jogging and exercise programs that given the proper opportunities, many will select health-related activities.

Applied psychology can now play a larger role in improving health care systems, testing methods, and instruments, particularly in the areas of the maintenance of health in old age, the packaging of consumer information and therapy, e.g., age specific approaches to sexual counseling, and the control of problems of polypharmacy. Psychological "problems" in old age are frequently linked to medical problems and therapies need to be placed in this context.

Elderly persons, relative to young adults, have greater needs for both acute and nonacute medical services, but the major difference in need stems from the greater incidence of chronic, or partially disabling medical or psychiatric problems. Usually the optimal treatment for such problems involves a mix of medical and social services geared toward maintaining the maximum degree of independence.

A major theme of the 1961, 1971 and the forthcoming 1981 White House Conferences on Aging concerns the development of social and medical programs which will further the goal of independent or noninstitutional living for the elderly. The 1978 amendments to the Older Americans Act as well as Administration on Aging (AOA) initiatives with its discretionary funds place considerable emphasis on developing programs of long-term care for the frail elderly based on these principles.

The desire for maintenance of continuity of an independent lifestyle and a repugnance for institutional living are frequently cited as motives for development of these programs. A description of the conditions under which such motives are valid requires more careful examination than received heretofore. For the widowed, partially disabled, isolated, impoverished elderly person, maintenance of independence in living arrangement may not be an optimal mode of living with respect to health or happiness because the physical independence gained may be at considerable psychological cost in companionship and comfort.

The personal, social as well as monetary costs of maintaining a sick elderly person at home or in the home of an adult child may be greater than we care to consider. With respect to economics, a recent U.S. General Accounting Office (1977) study showed that the costs of personal and medical services required to maintain a person at home increase very rapidly as the degree of disability increases. The level of disability at which such care was economical in the study was such that only 13% of the partially disabled elderly could be cared for at home at a cost less than that of institutionalization. The cut in earning power of an adult caregiver such as a daughter must also be considered in the cost of care, to say nothing of the well-being of the care giver.

One basis for planning the mix of required medical and social services for elderly persons is the classification of needs according to disability. Several such schemes have been devised by Williams, Bergner, Hill, Knox, and Fairbank (1973), a team of workers at Duke University (Pfeiffer 1977) and by Dr. Ralph Goldman for the Veterans Administration (Veterans Administration 1977). The unifying concept of all of these plans is the notion of a continuity of needs according to levels of disabilities which cut across a variety of specific diseases or illnesses.

Table 1.   Requirements for Services and Alternative Placement for Nine Levels of Disability

| Disability | Services Requirements | | | | Placement Alternatives | | | |
	Medical	Professional Nursing	Other^a	Non-Professional^b	Independent Home	Home/w Assistance	Nursing Home	Hospital
None	0	0	0	0	X			
Minimal	0/1	0	0	0	X	X		
Mild	0/1	0	0/1	0/	X	X		
Moderate	1	0/1	0/1	1/2		X	X	
Moderate Severe	1	1	0/1	2/3		X	X	
Severe Chronic Stable	1/2	0/1	0/1	3		X	X	
Severe Chronic Unstable	1/2	1/2	0/2	2/3				X
Acute Diagnostic	2/3	0/2	1/2	1/3				X
Severe Acute	3	3	2	1/2				X

Ratings: 0 = none or occasional as needed;   1 = monthly to weekly;   2 = daily;   3 = continuous (including intensive care)
a — physical therapy, rehabilitation therapy, inhalation therapy, etc.
b — home health aide, practical nurse, homemaker services, aids with shopping, activities of daily living.

Table 1 adapted from *The Aging Veteran* (Veterans Administration 1977) displays a nine-level classification of disability and indicates the typical needs for medical, nursing, nonprofessional and specialized assistance required at each level as well as typical alternative placements.

From the table it is clear that for six of the nine levels hospital care is not required, and that skilled or intermediate nursing home care is an appropriate placement for only three levels. Home or home with assistance is a theoretically acceptable alternative for a majority of levels of disability. The practicality of home care varies according to the resources available particularly a willing and able caretaker.

Psychological interventions at the various levels of disability shown in Table 1 can range from assisting individuals to adapt to severe disabilities in a hospital to rehabilitation efforts in long-term care settings (nursing homes) to the use of individual therapy of groups and peer support to foster a "satisfying" life at home. Perhaps more important psychologists can contribute to the recognition of the necessity of properly linking treatments to the needs of people.

The levels of disability discussed in Table 1 provide a restrictive view of the problem of long-term care. As pointed out by Lee and Estes (1979),

> Efforts to improve long-term care services via professionalization, medicalization, regulation, or the introduction of alternatives to nursing homes will not reach the problems of the aged. . . . If the current development continues. . . services will remain marginal in their capacity either to improve the lives of the aged or to reduce the escalating economic cost. This is because *these policies treat the problems of the aged as independent of the social causes,* while positing solutions involving the consumption of services (pp. 12-13). (emphasis added)

WORK AND LEISURE

In the surveys of the concerns of older persons, economic security and good health care are put at the top of the list. Older people want the good health and means to be able to maintain their style of life. Retirement for many people means a very substantial loss of income and status, and a void in their accustomed pattern of activities which now must be replaced with other time-filling activities, perhaps not as meaningful to them as work. From a developmental perspective the three topics are clearly interrelated. Leisure activites stereotypically supplant work in retirement and good health is critical to both.

The loss of relationships, resources, and roles is indeed an unfortunate aspect of aging, perhaps more so for those retiring from work than for those who have been at home all along. To successfully cope with these problems, planning for optimal person-environment interactions over the entire adult life span is required.

Work

Substantial progress has been made in overcoming barriers to older persons' working. Belbin and Belbin (1968) have pioneered the area of retraining older workers for new careers and in changed production methods which now may change frequently in the working life of one person. Current legislation has removed mandatory retirement age for Federal employees and raised the retirement age to seventy in the private sector.

Yet the right to continue working has not changed retirement practices noticeably. After reviewing a variety of data Monk and Donovan (1979) conclude that a threefold pattern will evolve: "The present trend toward early retirement (sixty to sixty-two) will continue as large numbers of workers begin drawing income supports from private pensions; second, conventional retirement will probably attract financially timid or cautious workers; and third, late retirement at seventy will appeal to achievement-oriented workers."

Monk and Donovan (1979) cite six requirements for a comprehensive retirement planning program including counseling or group activity starting part-time years prior to retirement and coverage of personal finances, health, housing, leisure and legal aspects. The review concludes that comprehensive retirement planning reaches less than 10% of the labor force. The review contains a number of excellent suggestions for needed research based on evidence from current practice. The tenor of the recommendations made by the writers makes it clear that the basis for helping persons adapt to retirement must emphasize the continuities of life after retirement as well as the obvious differences.

The literature cited on retirement planning raises the question of motivation for work. An excellent essay on the issue of common sense conceptions relative to the motivation for retirement and for work is given by Stearns (1979). Its value is considerable for providing a broad perspective to the issue for psychologists.

What about people who work only because they feel they have nothing else to do, or who hang on to a job because they literally can't afford to give it up? The fact that the removal of restrictions on the mandatory retirement age has affected retirement little makes us realize that work needs to be more satisfying throughout the adult years. The problems are vividly illustrated in the profession of engineering, a field which changes rapidly enough so that Dubin, Shelton, and McConnell (1974) estimate the half life of the usefulness of an engineer's formal training to be less than a decade.

In a conference called "Maintaining the Technical Competence of the Older Engineer," (Dublin, Shelton, McConnell 1974) the writer made several recommendations. To employers of engineers, the writer recommended that planning for long-term employment of engineers should incorporate portable pensions and other fiscal arrangements to promote mobility and change. Continuing education as a basis for maintaining a job was the last of the priorities (Fozard 1974).

For employees, the writer recommended using counseling and systematic planning for flexible payment schedules, a better balance between work and play, and other courses of action that would prepare one to deal with the predictable changes in life. It is clear that achieving these objectives—which are still thoroughly applicable at the present writing—involves more active intervention in people and the social aspects of their work environments.

Related to the above ideas is Miller's (1977) work on vitality. Miller argues that it is necessary to experience changes of interest within a career and changes in other non-work-related activitiy in order to have work be a significant determinant of one's morale and a significant factor in one's psychological well-being throughout the working career. According to Miller (and certainly according to Levinson as well) an inflexible career is detrimental to the mental health of an individual, and Miller provides a comprehensive set of recommendations for employees and employers relative to the maintenance of vitality. Several possibilities for job redesign relative to the maintenance of interest in work by engineers were suggested by Davis (1974) and Susman (1974) in the proceedings of the conference organized by Dubin, Shelton, and McConnell (1974).

The classic instrument relating occupational choice to interest patterns has been the Strong Vocational Interest Blank (Strong 1943). There is now evidence that the pattern of interests measured by the Strong Vocational Interest Blank is very stable over age (Campbell and Holland 1972; Costa, Fozard, and McCrae 1977). Moreover, the interest patterns measured in the instrument are related to enduring personality characteristics (Costa, Fozard, and McCrae 1977).

Levinson and his colleagues (Levinson et al. 1974) found that individuals who have previously worked very hard to internalize the values of their culture and succeed at their work now question the value and meaning of that work to themselves. This self-challenging of the importance and significance of work is not peculiar to particular occupations. The message from Levinson's work is straightforward; psychological counseling relative to the significance and importance of work should be part of one's experience.

Removal of formal age barriers to maintaining employment has increased the longstanding need for improving functional assessments of abilities and interests relative to maintenance of particular jobs. Concurrently, there has also been an increasing number of questions about the maximum age of initiating new jobs. The relationship of age changes in ability to acquire or keep a job is an issue charged with emotional overtones. The increasing use of the courts in cases involving age discrimination in employment has not resulted in greater clarification of the issues.

Despite the increased risk of litigation surrounding the use of ability tests in employment, the obligation to develop validated measures of aptitude is incumbent on psychologists.

The severity of the problems of age differences in ability as related to ability to work has probably been exaggerated. Research results and case studies indicate that abilities as well as a supposed reluctance to change are not uniformly greater barriers to older than to younger workers. Following World War II, European countries, China and Japan were faced with a devastated industrial capacity and a work force containing an abnormally high proportion of young and elderly workers. In many studies (e.g., Welford 1958) it was found that older workers adapted very well to changed production methods. However, in many cases the preferred method of training new skills was age-specific (Belbin and Belbin 1968). The issue relating ability to work to age is discussed more fully by Welford (1977) and Fozard and Popkin (1978).

Gerathewohl (1978a, b) explored the concept of functional age as it applied to pilot performance. From the literature he developed a taxonomy of performance (Gerathewohol 1978b) and recommended measuring pilot performance on the basis of automated records of aircraft performance such as magnetic heading, radio altimeter, glide slope deviations, etc. Gerathewohl outlines a seven-point developmental program which would relate automated flight performance data to assessments of pilot performance which he believes will ''. . .be useful not only for measuring pilot performance at a particular point in time but also for predicting later or expected proficiency through the analysis of current performance and its comparison with past performance.'' (Gerathewohl 1978b, p. 45-46) The detailed applied research needs to be performed.

There are very few, if any, occupations in which the technical capability for detailed assessment of an individual's performance is as highly developed as in piloting an aircraft. However, because of the relaxation of mandatory retirement rules as well as the increase in the interest and need for changing careers at older ages, the need for relating performance to employment creates a demand for improved psychological assessments of performance and aptitude that is greater than ever before.

Leisure

In contrast to work and health which impose restraints on behavior, leisure, in theory, allows one to exercise the maximum range of choices of activities. In recent years, there has been an increase in the range of sports equipment and consumer products for leisure activities. But the availability of such equipment is not directly related to the needs or interests of adults. From a developmental view, what is needed is much greater planning with respect to the choice of leisure activities over the life span. In adulthood, leisure is typically associated with retirement from work, but it is unwise to maintain such a restrictive attitude.

Gordon and Gaitz (1977) employed a two-dimensional classification system to analyze age differences in leisure activities. One dimension involves differences in level of activity ranging from passive and sedentary to vigorous and sensation-seeking. The other is a typology of activities including distinctions among noncompetitive and competitive sports, solitary versus group activities, and so on. The writers conclude that with increasing age, the level of activity decreases and the number of passive, solitary activities increases—all this despite greater opportunities for leisure activities in retirement. Satisfaction with low levels of activity is less among elder adults than with those who report relatively higher levels of activity and social involvement. However, the greater satisfaction of more activity is achieved at the cost of greater concern over the perceived risks of such activity.

Fozard and Popkin (1978) reported data consistant with both the findings and interpretations of Gordon and Gaitz (1977). In addition to rating present level of involvement in several classes of activities, subjects rated their anticipated level of involvement in retirement. Both cross-sectional (Fozard and Popkin 1978) and longitudinal findings (Fozard 1980) indicated that men consistently overestimate the degree of involvement following retirement in all classes of activities except reading and watching television.

With respect to mental health, physical health, adjustment, retirement, and so on, it is necessary to plan leisure activities that complement as well as supplement work and family roles which occupy much of middle age. This entails devising alternatives for those sports suitable only for the young who have leisure and strength for them, ones that are suitable for middle aged and older persons. As suggested by Miller (1977) promoting activities that balance work and play will do much to maintain stamina, a sense of well-being, and social activity over the lifespan.

Of practical interest, Fozard and Popkin (1978) reported results of multiple regression analyses performed on self-ratings of present and projected involvement in physical, solitary, social, and cultural activities. The independent variables in each analysis were three ability scores (Costa, Fozard, McCrae, and Bosse 1976), the five factor scores derived from the Strong Vocational Interest Blank (Costa, Fozard, and McCrae 1977), and chronological age at the time of responding to the questions on activities. Although statistically significant beyond the .01 level, the total amount of variance in the activity scores accounted for by these variables was small. Greater present involvement in physical activity was associated with higher verbal abilities, a stronger orientation toward people, greater orientation toward the helping professions, and age. Greater involvement with cultural events was associated with a more theoretical style of interaction, tender-mindedness, and greater extraversion.

Age was not a very powerful predictor of involvement in leisure activities when other, more meaningful psychological descriptors of an individual were included. Although the total variance accounted for by all of the variables was low, the results indicate that counseling relative to choices in work and leisure activities is practical especially if measurement of the criterion variables were improved.

At a more practical time Weiss' (1979) leisure planning program which relates six classes of problems, isolation and discontinuity, e.g., to a person's needs and goals can serve as a basis for a structural interview and is self-interpreting to the respondent.

MEMORY AND COGNITION

Fozard (1980) and Fozard and Popkin (1978) presented a proposal for intervention into memory problems of the elderly based on linking observed data on age deficits in capacity and efficiency of memory to variation in personality, motivation, and abilities. Possibilities for intervention include pharmacological (Hines and Fozard, in press) task redesign (Fozard 1980, in press) capitalizing on individual differences in personality and interests (Fozard and Costa, in press; Costa and Fozard 1978), and skill training (Poon, in press; Poon, Fozard, and Walsh-Sweeney 1980).

The analysis by Fozard (1980 pp. 283-284) argues that although further development is needed, clinical intervention is practical. Memory problems are one of the few mental health problems acknowledged as "respectable" by today's elderly. Therefore, the clincial treatment of this can have both direct and indirect mental health benefits. A program of intervention for memory problems of the elderly—including cognitive skill training, individual counseling, and the redesign of tasks—will reduce present limitation in our knowledge in at least four areas: (1) the interrelation in information obtained from formal assessments of memory and from problems of learning and memory in everyday life; (2) psychological assessments of memory and clinical procedures; (3) the potential for general ability and maintenance of cognitive skill training; and (4) responses of depression and transient emotional states to "normal age-related problems." (Fozard 1980, p. 283)

With respect to diagnosis, it is difficult to establish a clear relation between self-reported complaints and memory functions (Erickson 1978; Erickson and Scott 1977). Kahn and his associates (see Kahn and Miller 1978, for a review) have shown that elderly persons who manifest symptoms of depression are more likely to complain of memory problems than are nondepressed age peers with organic impairment as defined by behavioral assessments. However, Zelinski, Gilewski, and Thompson (1980) have described an improved self-report instrument that helps the respondent to define the situations in which memory problems occur and to describe the steps normally taken to deal with them. With this instrument Zelinski et al. found that older adults are much better at identifying problems than previously believed.

The treatment part of an intervention program should include cognitive skill training and counseling or psychotherapy (group and/or individual). Goals of the latter include providing motivation for acquiring and applying techniques embodied in cognitive skill training and for applying general techniques to specific problems. Another set of goals is to treat anxiety and/or depression and poor self-images that may be the result or the cause of memory complaints. The auxiliary treatment consists of treating medical problems that may contribute to the memory problem.

''Memory is a means to an end as well as an end in itself.'' (Hultsch and Pentz 1980). Since Freud's (1914/1956) classic description, it has been recognized that the phenomena of selectivity and motivation in remembering are at the core of most psychological diagnostic and treatment procedures and most everyday experiences of changes in memory. For the elderly the observation of a positive relation between reminiscing and adjustment has been at the core of a great deal of clinical theory and practice (Pfeiffer 1977), Butler's (1963) work on life review, or reconstruction of the past, being just one example. Partly as a reaction to the limitations of reality orientation for confused institutionalized elderly persons, Naomi Feil at the Cleveland Montefiore Home for the Aged has a devised a therapy to help elderly persons use the remnants of the past to achieve meaningful existence in their last years. The ideas are presented in the film *Looking for Yesterday,* in which the aged recall their past and integrate it into their lives.

An empirically based psychological analysis of the usefulness of and satisfaction with memory in old age is long overdue. The work of Giambra (1979) on age differences in daydreaming shows how content of motivational material differs with age. There are many implications for clinical practice and research in his findings.

How motivational differences related to memory and work is examined by Simone de Beauvoir in *The Coming of Age* (1972). She gives examples which illustrate how the accumulation of experience may hinder the successful pursuit of careers by trapping people in outmoded ways of thinking and desire to protect their accomplishments rather than to progress. Scientists appear particularly vulnerable to being trapped by their own past work, sometimes twisting facts to support their own outdated theories. The weakness of the scientist may be the strength of the writer or philosopher, who works with a more self-contained, imaginary intellectual system.

Painters and composers are also less susceptible to being victims of their own pasts.

Little is known about aging and memory in nonoccupational pursuits. Indirect evidence relating interests and age (Fozard and Popkin 1978; Fozard 1980) suggests that expectations for the future are a function of memory of past experiences in nonoccupational pursuits as well as in work. Their analyses are consistent with everyday expectations that memory as a tool in future plans and hopes can be deceptive. An empirical analysis of the issue is overdue and it should be an exciting one for psychology in the next decade.

PERCEPTION

Age-related perceptual losses in vision, hearing, and other sense modalities not only limit the range of behavior possibilities for an affected individual but may also markedly affect self-esteem and motivation for social interaction. A mix of counseling, training, and environmental intervention may do a great deal in itself to help an elderly person but may also set the stage for carrying out other more complex therapeutic interventions because of rapport established between therapist and client. The following is abstracted from Fozard (in press) and Fozard and Popkin (1978, pp 978-980).

Vision

The illumination required for satisfactory visual functioning increases with age, partly because of a greater scattering of light in the occular media, shrinking of the pupils, yellowing of the lens, and loss of accommodation. The age-related problems in visual functioning are different at various levels of illumination (Fozard et al. 1977).

Age differences in sensitivity to light at low levels of illumination were documented in a study of dark adaptation by Domey, McFarland, and Chadwick (1960) who found that after adaptation was complete, 240 times as much light was, on the average, required by a person in the oldest group as one in the youngest group to see the same target. The practical significance of the data lies in tasks which require partial rather than complete dark adaptation, i.e., a range of twilight illumination levels that require crossing between cone and rod vision. The terminal level of adaptation of the cone cells defines the time period when three-dimensional vision, acuity, and color vision cease, and the time before the rod cells have attained any useful degree of sensitivity.

The profound effect of age on the difficulty of reading traffic signs under low levels of illumination is described by Sivak, Olson, and Pastalan (in press).

At the other extreme, Wolf (1960) studied age in relation to very high levels of illumination and found that persons in their seventies required almost 100 times as much illumination as those in their twenties to detect targets in the presence of veiling glare. The extent of the practical difficulties resulting from glare are not well appreciated by the laiety, and the effects of glare on the acuity of older persons are seldom tested by the ophthamologist or optometrist. Pastalan et al. (1973) suggest that many older individuals who have adequate acuity and depth perception under the conditions common in drivers's tests will be greatly handicapped in reading road signs in bright daylight.

Studies of office productivity show that in the middle levels of illumination, there are also important age differences in visibility. Guth, Eastman, and McNeils (1956) measured the contrast needed by individuals in different age groups to attain the same visual performance as that of the average twenty-year old. The requisite levels increased dramatically in subjects over seventy. More recently Hughes (1977) verified and extended these results.

The above findings indicate that manipulating levels of illumination can compensate for many of the visual problems of the elderly. Work spaces and living areas should be planned so that individual differences in illumination requirements can be accommodated. Older persons are likelier to need more local light on work areas rather than the entire surroundings. Contrast in visual information displays should be maximized as on labels of bottles and the information on the switches and control panels of household appliances. Local lighting of steps and ramps may counter the adverse effects of age-related slowing of dark and light adaptation and sensitivity to glare which handicap the older persons's mobility under low levels of illumination and abrupt changes therein.

Relatively little work has been performed on training older persons in perceptual tasks since the classic research described by Welford (1958). A training task for the elderly driver has been described recently by Sterns, Barrett, and Alexander (1977). The training was based on the belief that automotive accidents are related in part to idiosyncratic problems in perceptual style, selective attention, and variations in perceptual-motor reaction patterns. The results indicated that while training increased the general information processing skills of elderly drivers, the relationship between performance on the tasks and actual driving needs further investigation.

The findings make it clear that there is a great need for improvement in functional tests for tasks such as driving. Increasing the frequency of visual screening tests for older persons as is the pattern in memory studies will be of little value unless the tests assess the problems unique to the aged. In our increasingly litigious society there could be a basis for legal action against licensing bodies which persist in using tests that don't identify the major problems of older drivers. A start in improving this situation has been made with the development of a visual testing battery described by Shinar (1977). Significantly, these issues are not addressed in the conventional tests of visual function.

Audition

The literature cited under the section on vision provides many examples of how the dependence of behavior on information from the environment is greater with older age. Audition provides a similar spectrum of examples (See Corso 1977 for a review). Most importantly, presbycusis causes problems in speech perception that are not always predictable from pure tone audiometry.

The implications of research reviewed by Corso (1977) and Fozard (in press) are that the range of broad environmental manipulations of the auditory signal with respect to background loudness that will specifically aid the elderly is somewhat limited. For example, improvement of the quality of public address systems to a level marginally acceptable to younger adults will probably not be as helpful for older persons. Similarly, hearing aids provide relief for only some of the auditory problems of the elderly.

Relatively greater reliance on training of interpersonal and social skills are necessary in order to help older persons overcome common auditory difficulties than is the case in vision. An instructive anecdote was told by Dr. Oliver Welsh, Chief of Audiology at the Veterans Administration Outpatient Clinic, Boston, concerning a veteran patient who incorrectly attributed a supposed hearing loss to his age. Testing revealed no loss that required a hearing aid. The history indicated that since his military discharge the veteran changed his employment from construction worker to lawyer, a change from an occupation in which speech perception and understanding was relatively less important to one where it was crucial. Thus, a mild defect became important. Therapy consisted of training the veteran to overcome his fear to ask that information to be repeated, to seat himself advantageously in groups and to use other skills to improve his auditory perception.

The example illustrates many practical issues that must be faced by older persons who do not want to embarrass themselves by appearing not to understand speech. Corso (1977) concluded that there is a great deal of applied work to be done in this area.

Taste, Smell and Dental Prostheses

The relatively sparse literature on age differences in perceptual thresholds for taste and smell have been summarized by Engen (1977). Recent research has shown that apparent age-related differences in taste and food preference are more directly related to the use of partial and complete dentures than to age as such (House, Rissin, and Kapur 1977).

The practical implications of the research summarized by Chauncey and House (1979) are clear: the use of partial over complete dentures should be encouraged whenever possible; dentures should be replaced periodically; physicians should also include an evaluation of periodontal disease in their elderly patients (Chauncy and House 1977). The importance of the role of counseling in the adaptation to and proper use of dentures is stressed by these writers.

The common theme throughout the section on perception is that psychologists have a role in improving consumer acceptance of sensory prostheses, direct skill training, as well as counseling on adaptation to perceptual difficulties.

PROFESSIONAL CONSIDERATIONS

A recent analysis of personnel needs for psychologists in the field of gerontology, Fozard (1977) devoted over 60% of the space to clinical, counseling, and engineering psychologists because these occupational specialities represent the groups for which the greatest potential for utilization lies. The article recognized the differences between projected need and job availability and suggested that the acceptability of psychologists in the roles described would have to be won. In particular, it is recognized that clinical psychologists have, except for neuropsychological assessment, moved away from psychological evaluations in favor of psychotherapy and that they, like other psychotherapists have avoided working with the elderly. As a result, social workers and nonprofessionals (as in the Ypsilante Hospital experience) have taken over many of the traditional treatment roles.

The psychologist can establish a unique role with the elderly by bringing all his research and clinical training and a transactional view of adult development to bear on psychogerontology. His ability to conceptualize the relative roles of psychotherapy and environmental intervention in the treatment of the elderly is unique. However, it requires the typical applied psychologist to think beyond his own specialty.

The present chapter has identified several areas of emphasis for applied psychology. Clinicians and counselors are perhaps more accustomed to defining target populations. From such a view, the elderly with mental illness may be classified as institutionalized and diagnosed, noninstitutionalized and diagnosed, nondiagnosed, and at risk. For each subpopulation the potential range of useful psychological interventions differs. The present article has focussed on the most ''normal'' groups because of a desire to stress the normal age-related differences and variations in behavior that potentially affect clinical practice.

References

Baltes, P. B., & Willis, S. L. Toward psychological theories of aging and development. In J. E. Birren & K. W. Schaie (eds.), *Handbook of the psychology of aging.* New York: Van Nostrand Reinhold, 1977.

Belbin, E., & Belbin, R. M. New careers in middle age. In B. Neugarten (ed.), *Middle age and aging: A reader in social psychology.* Chicago: University of Chicago Press, 1968.

Blenker, M. Environmental change and the aging individual. *Gerontologist,* 1967, *7:* 101-105.

Butler, R. N. The life review: An interpretation of reminiscence in the aged. *Psychiatry,* 1963, *26:* 65-76.

Campbell, D. P., & Holland, J. L. A merger in vocational interest research: applying Holland's theory to Strong's data. *Journal of Vocational Behavior,* 1972, *2:* 353-376.

Chauncey, H. H., & House, J. E. Dental problems of the elderly. *Hospital Practice,* 1977,*12:* 81-86.

Corso, J. F. Auditory perception and communication. In J. E. Birren & K. W. Schaie (eds.), *Handbook of the psychology of aging.* New York: Van Nostrand Reinhold, 1977.

Costa, P. T., & Fozard, J. L. Remembering the person: relations of individual difference variables to memory. *Experimental Aging Research,* 1978, *4:* 291-304.

Costa, P. T., Fozard, J. L., & McCrae, R. R. Personological interpretation of factors from the Strong Vocational Interest Blank scales. *Journal of Vocational Behavior,* 1977, *10:* 231-243.

Costa, P. T., Fozard, J. L., McCrae, R. R., & Bosse, R. Relations of age and personality dimensions to cognitive ability factors. *Journal of Gerontology,* 1976, *31:* 663-669.

Costa, P. T., & McCrae, R. R. Age differences in personality structure: A cluster analytic approach. *Journal of Gerontology,* 1976, *31:* 564-570.

Davis, L. W. Design of jobs. In S. S. Dubin, H. Shelton, & J. McConnell (eds.), *Maintaining professional and technical competence of the older engineer.* Washington, D.C.: American Society for Engineering Education, 1974.

deBeauvoir, S. *Coming of age.* (translated by Patrick O'Brian). New York: Putnam's, 1972.

Domey, R. C., McFarland, R. A., & Chadwick, E. Dark adaptation as a function of age and time: II. A derivation. *Journal of Gerontology,* 1960, *15:* 267-279.

Dowd, J. J. Exchange rates and old people. *Journal of Gerontology,* 1980, *35:* 596-601.

Dubin, S. S., Shelton, H., & McConnel, J. (eds.) *Maintaining professional and technical competence of the older engineer.* Washington, D.C.: American Society for Engineering Education, 1974.

Engen, T. Taste and smell. In J. E. Birren & K. W. Schaie (eds.), *Handbook of the psychology of aging.* New York: Van Nostrand Reinhold, 1977, 554-561.

Erickson, R. C., & Scott, M. L. Clinical memory testing: A review. *Psychological Bulletin,* 1977, *84:* 1130-1149.

Fozard, J. L. Changing person-environment relationships in adulthood. *Human Factors,* in press.

Fozard, J. L. Facts and fiction about behavior changes with age: Implications for the concepts of obsolescence and vitality as applied to the engineer. In S. S. Dubin, H. Shelton, & J. McConnell (eds.), *Maintaining professional and technical competence of the older engineer,* pp. 55-71. Washington, D.C.: American Society for Engineering Education, 1974.

Fozard, J. L. Life begins at 30: training and employment opportunities in the psychology of aging. *Educational Gerontology,* 1977, *3:* 351-357.

Fozard, J. L. The time for remembering. In L. W. Poon (ed.), *Aging in the 1980s: Selected contemporary issues in the psychology of aging.* Washington, D.C.: American Psychological Association, 1980.

Fozard, J. L., & Costa, P. T. Age differences in memory and decision making in relation to personality, abilities, and endocrine function: Implication for clinical practice and health planning policy. In M. Mairos (ed.), *Proceedings, aging: a challenge for science and social policy.* London: Oxford University, in press.

Fozard, J. L., & Popkin, S. J. Optimizing adult development: Ends and means of an applied psychology of aging. *American Psychologist,* 1978, *33:* 975-989.

Fozard, J. L., & Thomas, J. C. Psychology of aging: basic findings and some practical implications. In J. G. Howells (ed.), *Modern perspectives in the psychology of old age.* New York: Brunner/Mazel, 1975.

Fozard, J. L., Wolf, E., Bell, B., McFarland, R. A., & Podolsky, S. Visual perception and communication. In J. E. Birren & K. W. Schaie (eds.), *Handbook of the psychology of aging.* New York: Van Nostrand Reinhold, 1977.

Freud, S. The psychopathology of everyday life. In A. A. Brill (ed.), *The basic writings of Sigmund Freud,* Vol. IV. London: Hogarth, 1956.

Gerathewohl, S. J. Psychophysiological effects of aging—developing a functional age index for pilots: II. Taxonomy of psychological factors, Office of Aviation Medicine, Federal Aviation Administration, Report FAA-AM-78-16, March 1978.

Gerathewohl. S. J. Psychophysiological effects of aging—developing a functional age index for pilots: III. Measurement of pilot performance. Office of Aviation Medicine, Federal Aviation Administration, Report FAA-AM-78-27, August 1978.

Giambra, L. M. Sex differences in daydreaming and related mental activity from the late teens to the early nineties. *Aging and Human Development,* 1979, *10:* 1-34.

Gordon, C., & Gaitz, C. M. Leisure and lives: personal expressivity across the life span. In R. H. Binstock & E. Shanas (eds.), *Handbook of aging and the social sciences.* New York: Van Nostrand Reinhold, 1977.

Guth, S. K., Eastman, A. A., & McNelis, J. F. Lighting requirements for older workers. *Illumination Engineering,* 1956: *30:* 307-311.

Hines, T. M., & Fozard, J. L. Memory and aging: Relevance of recent developments for research and application. In C. Eisdorfer (ed.), *Annual Review of Gerontology and Geriatrics,* Vol. I. New York: Springer, in press.

House, J. E., Rissin, L., & Kapur, K. K. Analysis of the interrelationship between masticatory performance and food preference. *Journal of Dental Research* (Special Issue B), 1977, *56:* 236.

Hughes, P. C. The contribution of lighting to productivity and quality of work life. Paper presented at the meeting of the Institute of Electrical and Electronics Engineers, Industry Applications Society, Los Angles, June 1977.

Hultsch, D. F., & Pentz, C. A. Encoding, storage, and retrieval in adult memory: The role of model assumptions. In L. W. Poon, J. L. Fozard, L. S. Cermak, D. Arenberg, & L. W. Thompson (eds.), *New directions in memory and aging: Proceedings of the George A. Talland Memorial Conference.* Hillsdale, N.J.: Lawrence Erlbaum, 1980.

Kahn, R. L., and Miller, N. E. Adaptational factors in memory function in the aged. *Experimental Aging Research,* 1978, *4:* 273-290.

Lawton, M. P., & Nahemow, L. Ecology and the aging process. In C. Eisdorfer & M. P. Lawton (eds.), *The psychology of adult development and aging.* Washington, D.C.: American Psychological Association, 1973.

Lee, P. R., & Estes, C. L. Public policies, the aged, and long-term care. *The Journal of Long-Term Care Administration,* 1979, November: 1-15.

Levinson, D. J., Darrow, C. M., Klein, E. B., Levinson, M. D., & McKee, B. The psychosocial development of men in early adulthood and the mid-life transition. In D. F. Ricks, A. Thomas, & M. Roff (eds.), *Life history research in psychopathology* (Vol. 3). Minneapolis: University of Minnesota Press, 1974.

Miller, D. *Personal vitality.* Reading, Mass.: Addison-Wesley, 1977.

Monk, A., & Donovan, R. Pre-retirement preparation programs. *Aged Care and Services Review,* 1978-1979, *1:* (5-6), *1,* 3-7.

Moos, R., & Houts, P. The assessment of the social atmosphere of psychiatric wards. *Journal of Abnormal Psychology,* 1968, *73:* 595-604.

Moos, R. H., & Lemke, S. Assessing the physical and architectural features of sheltered care settings. *Journal of Gerontology,* 1980, *35:* 584-595.

Moos, R., Shelton, R., & Petty, C. Perceived ward climate and treatment outcome. *Journal of Abnormal Psychology,* 1973, *82:* 291-298.

Neugarten, B. L. Introduction to the symposium "Models and Methods for the Study of the Life Cycle," *Human Development,* 1971, *14:* 81-86.

Pastalan, L. A., Mautz, R. K., & Merril, J. The simulation of age related losses: A new approach to the study of environmental barriers. In W. P. E. Preiser (ed.), *Environmental design research* (Vol. 1). Stroudsberg, Pa.: Powden, Hutchinson, & Ross, 1973.

Pfeiffer, E. Psychopathology and social pathology. In J. E. Birren & K. W. Schaie (eds.), *Handbook of the psychology of aging.* New York: Van Nostrand Reinhold, 1977.

Poon, L. W. A systems approach for the assessment and treatment of memory problems. In J. Ferguson & C. B. Taylor (eds.), *Advances in behavioral medicine.* New York: Spectrum Press, in press.

Poon, L. W., Fozard, J. L., & Walsh-Sweeney, L. Memory training for the elderly: Salient issues on the use of imagery mnemonics. In L. W. Poon, J. L. Fozard, L. S. Cermak, D. Arenberg, & L. W. Thompson (eds.), *New directions in memory and aging: Proceedings of the George A. Talland Memorial Conference.* Hillsdale, N.J.: Lawrence Erlbaum, 1980.

Reigel, K. F. Adult life crisis: Toward a dialectic theory of development. In N. Daton & L. H. Ginsberg (eds.), *Life span development psychology: normative life crisis.* New York: Academic Press, 1975: 97-124.

Schaie, K. W., & Schaie, J. P. Clinical assessment and aging. In J. E. Birren & K. W. Schaie (eds.), *Handbook of the psychology of aging.* New York: Van Nostrand Reinhold, 1977.

Shinar, D. Driver visual limitations diagnosis and treatment. Final Report, Department of Transportation Contract, DOT-HS-5-1275, September 9, 1977, National Technical Information Service, Springfield, VA 22151.

Simon, J. R. Effects of age on the behavior of hospitalized patients. *Journal of Gerontology,* 1964, *19:* 364-369.

Sivak, M., Olson, P. L., & Pastalan, L. A. Effect of drivers' age on night time legibility of highway signs. *Human factors,* in press.

Spark, R. The case against regular physicals. *The New York Times Magazine,* July 25, 1976: pp. 10-11; 38-39.

Stearns, P. N. Future shock: the old folks version. *Perspective on Aging,* 1979, November/December: 11-17.

Sterns, H. L., Barrett, G. V., & Alexander, R. A. Training the older adult for effective driving performance. In J. L. Fozard (Chair) *Industrial gerontological psychology: Current research and issues.* Symposium presented at the meeting of the American Psychological Association, San Francisco, August 1977.

Strong, E. K., Jr. *Vocational interests of men and women.* Stanford, California: Stanford University Press, 1943.

Susman, G. I. Enriching the engineer's work role. In S. S. Dubin, H. Shelton, & J. McConnell (eds.), *Maintaining professional and technical competence of the older engineer.* Washington, D.C.: American Society for Engineering Education, 1974.

U.S. General Accounting Office. Condition of older people: National information system needed. Washington, D.C.: Report HRD-79-95, September 20, 1977.

Veterans Administration Central Office. *The aging veteran: Present and future medical needs* (Report submitted by the Chief Medical Director). Washington, D.C.: U.S. Government Printing Office, 1977.

Weiss, C. R. Leisure planning programs. *Perspective on Aging,* November/December, 1979: 18-22.

Welford, A. T. Motor performance. In J. E. Birren & K. W. Schaie (eds.), *Handbook of the psychology of aging.* New York: Van Nostrand Reinhold, 1977.

Welford, A. T. *Aging and human skill.* London: Oxford University Press, 1958.

Williams, T. F., Hill, J. G., Knox, K. G., & Fairbank, M. E. Appropriate placement of the chronically ill and aged. *Journal of the American Medical Association,* 1973, *226:* 1332-1335.

Wolf, E. Glare and age. *Archives of Ophthalmology,* 1960, *64:* 502-514.

Zelinski, E. M., Gilweski, M. J. & Thompson, L. W. Do laboratory memory tests relate to everyday remembering and forgetting? In L. W. Poon, J. L. Fozard, L. S. Cermak, D. Arenberg, & L. W. Thompson (eds.), *New directions in memory and aging: Proceedings of the George Talland Memorial Conference.* Hillsdale, N.J.: Lawrence Erlbaum, 1980.

Index

About the Contributors

SCOTT DANFORD is Associate Professor of Environmental Psychology in the School of Architecture and Environmental Design at the State University of New York at Buffalo.

Dr. Danford is an active author and researcher in the multidisciplinary field of Environment and Behavior with numerous publications in reseach methodology, environmental design education, and theory of person-environment relations.

Dr. Danford holds a Ph.D. in psychology from the University of Houston.

JAMES L. FOZARD, Ph.D., is the Director, Patient Treatment Service, of the Office of Extended Care, Veterans Administration, Washington, D.C. He is past president of the Division of Adult Development and Aging of the American Psychological Association and the Chairman of the Association's Task Force for the 1981 White House Conference on the Aging.

Dr. Fozard has written over sixty articles and chapters in the field of psychology of aging.

ARTHUR MACNEILL HORTON JR., is the Director of the Neuropsychology Laboratory at the Veterans Administration Medical Center in Martinsburg, West Virginia. He has held academic appointments at the University of Virginia and the Citadel, the Military College of South Carolina.

Dr. Horton has published and presented over sixty papers and articles. He has received numerous honors and awards for his work including a Dissertation Research Award from the University of Virginia and a Clinical Fellowship in the Behavior Therapy and Research Society.

Dr. Horton holds a B.A., M.Ed., and Ed.D. from the University of Virginia in Charlottesville, Virginia.

RONALD J. KARPF is Clinical Assistant Professor at Hahnemann Medical College and Hospital in Philadelphia. He is also Senior Clinical Psychologist at Eugenia Hospital in Whitemarsh, Pennsylvania.

Dr. Karpf is on the book review staff of the *American Journal of Psychotherapy*. He has published articles in the *Journal of General Psychology, Journal of Social Psychology, Psychotherapy: Theory, Research and Practice* and the *Journal of the American Geriatric Society*.

ROBERT W. KENNEDY, Ph.D., is a counseling psychologist whose clinical practice and research interests center on problems of aging.

ANN B. KENNEDY, Ph.D., is Assistant Professor of Special Education at Cabrini College, Radnor, Pennsylvania.

BRUCE B. KERR is a Ph.D. candidate in Clinical Psychology at the University of Massachusetts. He has done research in the processes underlying obesity and has co-authored several papers in that area.

Mr. Kerr is currently investigating responses to assertive behavior.

CHRISTINE A. LEWIS has been a speech pathologist and clinical supervisor with the Veterans Administration for eight years. She has been on the faculty of Metropolitan State College, Denver, Colorado, and is an Adjunct Instructor at West Virginia University.

Ms. Lewis has presented papers or workshops for the Clinical Aphasiology Conference, the Eastern Psychological Association, and the American Physical Therapy Association.

Ms. Lewis received an M.A. and a C.C.C. from California State University and is a certified member of the American Speech and Hearing Association.

MAURICE E. LINDEN is Professor of Psychiatry at Thomas Jefferson Medical School. Previously, he was Program Director of Gerontologic Study Center at Norristown, Pennsylvania State Hospital. He was also the founding fellow of the American College of Psychiatrists in 1963.

Dr. Linden pioneered the use of group therapy for geriatric patients and has published extensively, including the chapter "Geriatrics", in *The Fields of Group Psychotherapy,* edited by S.R. Slavson.

Dr. Linden received his medical degree from the University of California and is board certified in Psychiatry and Neurology.

MARIAN L. MACDONALD is currently Associate Professor of Psychology at the University of Massachusetts at Amherst. She has held previous appointments at the University of Illinois, the University of Hawaii, and the State University of New York at Stony Brook.

Dr. MacDonald is on the board of directors of the Association for Advancement of Behavior Therapy and has published extensively in the areas of behavior therapy, behavioral assessment and behavior modification with the aging.

GEORGE M. USOVA, Ph.D., is currently an education specialist in the U.S. Department of Education. Previously, he was Associate Professor of Education and Coordinator of the Graduate Reading Program at the Citadel.

Dr. Usova has authored over forty-five professional journal articles in the field of reading instruction and has recently published *Take Ten,* a reading series of fifty short stories for disabled readers.